ACHIEVING THE DOCTOR DREAM

THE COMPLETE GUIDE TO PREMEDICAL SUCCESS

GREGORY A. ANDREWS M.D. J.D. F.C.L.M.

PHYSICIAN AND ATTORNEY

FELLOW OF THE AMERICAN COLLEGE

OF LEGAL MEDICINE

MedLaw Books, Inc.
Erie, Pennsylvania

Publisher
MedLaw Books, Inc.
PO Box 4007
Erie, PA 16512-4007

Credits: A list of credits recognizing the companies which have books appearing on the cover of this publication can be found in the Acknowledgments Section.

Library of Congress Catalog Card Number: 97-092571

ISBN: 0-9660525-0-1

Printed in the United States of America

10 9 8 7 6 5 4 3 2 1

Dedication

To my parents

Thank you for your love, encouragement, and support.

To all patients who have touched my life

Helping to make a difference in your lives has made becoming a physician worth all of the time, effort, and sacrifice.

About the Author

Gregory A. Andrews M.D. J.D. F.C.L.M. is a graduate of Harvard University and received his Doctor of Medicine from the State University of New York at Buffalo School of Medicine and his Juris Doctorate from the University of Notre Dame Law School. He is a Fellow of the American College of Legal Medicine and has licenses to practice both medicine and law.

Contents

Preface

CONGRATULATIONS! If you are reading this book, you have already committed yourself, or at least have begun to think about a rewarding career in medicine. This is a "nuts and bolts" approach to succeeding in your premedical studies. It is a "tell it as it is" book about the realities of what it really means to be "premed." Each chapter is written for a variety of readers; whether you are in high school or a college undergraduate/graduate or a person without a degree going back to college, every chapter in this book contains valuable insights and information that is "user friendly." Parents, family members, and spouses of those committed to premedicine will also gain a good understanding "of what's really involved" in the process before one first attains the privilege of stepping into a medical school as a "student doctor." Though no "how to book" can absolutely guarantee success or admission, the insights contained in this book can carefully guide your premedical years and help you achieve your goal if you "truly want to become a doctor."

Gregory A. Andrews M.D. J.D. F.C.L.M.

Acknowledgments

I would like to thank the Association of American Medical Colleges for allowing me to use both sample application forms and other factual information which is cited in this book.

I am also grateful to the publishing companies which have given formal permission for their books to appear in the photographs on the cover of this publication. These books, along with their publishers, include the following: R. Finney and G. Thomas Jr., *Calculus,* 2nd Edition, ©1994, Addison-Wesley Longman Inc.; *Biology,* 4th Edition, by Neil A. Campbell, Copyright ©1996 by Benjamin/Cummings Publishing Company; Gabbe, Niebyl, and Simpson, *Obstetrics: Normal and Problem Pregnancies,* 3rd Edition, ©1996, Churchill Livingstone Inc.; Ebbing, Darrell D., *General Chemistry,* 5th Edition, Copyright ©1996 by Houghton Mifflin Company; Brinkley, *American History: A Survey,* 9th Edition, ©1995, McGraw-Hill, Inc.; Fauci et al. *Harrison's Principles of Internal Medicine,* 14th Edition, ©1998, McGraw-Hill, Inc.; Hardman et al. *Goodman and Gilman's The Pharmacological Basis of Therapeutics,* 9th Edition, ©1996, McGraw-Hill, Inc.; Schwartz et al. *Principles of Surgery.* 6th Edition. ©1994. New York, NY: McGraw-Hill, Inc.; Netter, M.D., Frank H. *Atlas of Human Anatomy,* ©1989, Novartis Pharmaceutical Corporation, Summit, NJ; Burns et al. *Government by the People,* 16th Edition, ©1995, Upper Saddle River, NJ: Prentice-Hall, Inc.; Morrison and Boyd, *Organic Chemistry,* 6th Edition, ©1992, Prentice-Hall, Inc.; Roberts and Jacobs, *Literature: An Introduction to Reading and Writing,* 5th Edition. ©1998, Prentice-Hall, Inc.; *Physics for Scientists and Engineers,* Fourth Edition, by Raymond A. Serway, Saunders College Publishing, Copyright ©1996 by Raymond A. Serway; Behrman et al. *Nelson Textbook of Pediatrics,* 15th Edition, ©1996, W.B. Saunders Company; Cotran, Kumar, and Robbins, *Robbins Pathologic Basis of Disease,* 5th Edition, ©1994, Philadelphia, PA: W.B. Saunders Company; Guyton and Hall, *Textbook of Medical Physiology.* 9th Edition, ©1996, Philadelphia, PA: W.B. Saunders Company.

I would like to recognize the dedication and hard work of Brenda Anderson who typed most of this manuscript. The secretarial assistance of Debbie Marsh and Susan Bennett is also appreciated.

I would also like to thank Susan Kellogg of Kellogg Design for helping with the book format and cover design. I am also grateful to Mr. James Leveson of Leveson Photography who did outstanding work on the cover photographs.

1
Introduction

Medical school admissions have undergone a major renaissance since the 1970s. Look at almost any medical school class nowadays and you will see a wide variety of ages, personal backgrounds, college majors, and racial and ethnic groups. "My daughter, the doctor" is now heard just as often as the traditional "my son, the doctor." Go to any medical school graduation and you will see children crowding around their newly degreed "doctor mom" or "doctor dad." As one can see, the personal makeup of the medical profession has indeed changed. It appears that medical schools will continue this "open door" policy regarding prospective applicants. Basically, you do not have to be a 21- or 22- year-old applicant anymore; "the sky really is the limit" nowadays when it comes to applying to medical school. Given this "open door" environment, premedical students must be aware that admission to medical school will continue to be extremely competitive.

Given our "uncertain economic environment," many students are placing "job security" as a top priority for their futures. Compared to any profession in today's world, the practice of medicine can provide that "job security." What's more important, however, is that the added benefits of being a doctor cannot be quantified: The ability to "make a difference"—to heal, to save lives, to promote good health maintenance—these factors make a physician's career most rewarding. As a medical school applicant, you can be sure that you have chosen the right profession.

Note, for example, that many students are "shying away" from formal business careers. Mergers, acquisitions, and corporate takeovers are cutting out thousands of middle management positions — positions that cannot be saved even if you possess an MBA or have years of experience or "company loyalty." The idea of serving a "corporate entity" has become less attractive to numerous students; "professional fulfillment" has been transformed into something of higher value. "Corporate loyalty" has been replaced by practicing a profession that AFFECTS PEOPLE'S LIVES DIRECTLY AND MAKES A DIFFERENCE!

If you are considering a premedical course, the following issues and questions should first be considered in your overall "premed plan" (These factors are the same whether you are a high school student, college student or graduate, or an older "non-traditional" applicant):

1. Do I have a true commitment to become a doctor? What does "it really take" to become one? How should I go about getting "health care experience" to gain insight into the medical profession?

2. What specific course requirements must I fulfill in order to apply to medical school?

3. Evaluation of your own academic strengths and weaknesses (especially in science and mathematics).

4. What type of premedical advisory services are available at my college?

5. How do I create a "general plan" to obtain admission into medical school two, three, or even four or more years down the road? What should my approach be in building a personal resumé?

ALL OF THESE ISSUES AND MUCH, MUCH MORE ARE COVERED IN THIS BOOK. The pathway to medical school really is a maze containing a myriad of questions all along the way. Getting answers to those questions and obtaining insight into what it "REALLY TAKES" TO GET INTO MEDICAL SCHOOL IS WHAT THIS BOOK IS ALL ABOUT!

Aspiring medical students will need to be aware of the challenges that will face them in the health care system. Some examples of these include the following:

1. ETHICAL DECISIONS AND CHOICES will remain one of the top challenges in medicine. Technological advances are moving "faster than the law," leaving doctors and their patients (and families) with major decisions that will affect people's lives and well-being. These issues cover the entire range of a person's life—from reproductive technologies to end-of-life ethical decisions.

2. MANAGED CARE (*e.g.* HMOs) has already become the "organization principle" for the way in which medicine is being practiced. Cost control (with "buzz words" like insurance authorization codes and utilization review) will continue to be the main emphasis as the "fee-for-service" approach has become a "practice of the past." The liberal use of tests and procedures has already been limited by the insurance industry; doctors will continuously face the challenge of insurance companies encroaching on their independence as medical practitioners.

3. PRIMARY CARE SPECIALTIES (*e.g.* general internal medicine, family practice, general pediatrics, and obstetrics and gynecology [primary care for women]) will continue to be of utmost importance in the health care system. The primary care practitioner provides both continuity of care along with preventive measures to reduce the incidence of chronic diseases.

These doctors also act as the "gatekeepers" in a managed care system: a referral to a specialist will depend on the primary care doctor's decision regarding the diagnosis and treatment of the medical (or potentially surgical) condition or disorder.

4. EMPHASIS ON THE EDUCATION OF PATIENTS

The prevention of disease will remain as a primary goal in our health care system. Counseling patients on principles such as weight control, diet, lifestyles, immunizations, decreasing potential cancer risks, is a prime method by which the quality of life can be greatly improved.

The public is also more well-informed about personal health care issues. Patients desire to be active participants in diagnostic and treatment decisions that will affect them. A person's understanding of a diagnostic test or therapeutic procedure means that a doctor must have the ability to communicate well with his/her patients.

5. THE PRACTICE OF MEDICINE ITSELF HAS UNDERGONE MAJOR CHANGES.

The health care team involves doctors, nurses, nurse practitioners, physician assistants, physical therapists, etc. This health care team approach is helping to improve the accessibility to comprehensive care and to control increasing medical costs.

There is also a great increase in the number of salaried physicians who are working in hospital, clinic, and managed care settings in order to establish or maintain a successful medical practice. Solo and two-person physician practices are "giving way" to larger group practices and even "multi-specialty" practices. Many doctors are also observing the fact that excellent practice opportunities exist in middle/smaller-size towns and rural areas.

It is really never too early or too late to plan your premedical education. Some students know that they TRULY want to be doctors since grade school or high school and develop their personal and academic credentials ("building their premed resumé") for a number of years. The very good news is that if you are not one of those students, you can still EXCEL in premed coursework, medical school, and in professional life. No matter what your education, background, or even "previous career," the road to success can be achieved if you remain disciplined, hard-working, and focused on your ultimate career goal. Remember, every college freshman class is filled with "doctor want-to-be's"—freshmen premeds who talked for years about how they were going to be doctors—only to drop their medical school plans after one or two semesters. What many of these students lacked is the TRUE DESIRE to become physicians; the formula for premedical success is one that will never fail the aspiring physician if it is taken seriously at an early stage in one's career.

The formula is as follows: CONSISTENCY + PERSISTENCY = SUCCESS; these two concepts not only involve the attributes of discipline and hard work but include the ability to AVOID PROCRASTINATION and to appreciate the meaning of "delayed gratification." The "formula for success" is introduced to show that the "doctor dream" can be achieved no matter what your academic background may be; if you TRULY want to become a doctor, that dream can be ACHIEVED!

2

Laying the Groundwork:
The First Building Blocks
for Premedical Success

Before formulating both your own plan for academic premedical coursework and for selecting a major, the following list of concepts is introduced to give you some guiding principles. Some of these concepts are discussed in detail in this chapter while others, along with their reference chapters, are analyzed elsewhere in this book.

1. <u>As a Student, You Must Learn to "Stay Within Yourself"</u>

You have to know your academic strengths and weaknesses even before you select your first semester premed courses. If you overextend yourself by taking too many difficult courses or a difficult course load too soon, your premed career may be over in just one or two semesters.

Some students make the mistake of "rushing through" their freshman year trying to complete half of their premed requirements. While some students are successful, others attempting to do this find themselves "out of" premed by the end of their freshman year. If you do not have a strong high school science or math background, you should concentrate on a more realistic class schedule. Just because all the other freshmen premeds on your dorm floor are taking calculus that first semester, doesn't mean that you should! If you have not had calculus in high school, it would benefit you to take college algebra/trigonometry (or a "pre-calculus" class) and do well in it. Getting an "A" in that first math course will help your science/math GPA for medical school admission and will also increase your confidence levels. Also, remember that having very good algebra/trigonometry skills are essential to doing well in calculus! A good foundation in algebra and trigonometry will also help you later when taking general physics.

In a similar manner, some students attempt to take classes that they SHOULD NOT— based on their initial academic performance; for example, if you received a "C" (or "just slipped by" with a "B") in a calculus class, it would not be a good idea to take calculus-based

---

physics (unless it was required for your major or program; if it is, you need to improve your performance and get extra tutorial help). Be aware that a medical school admissions committee would rather see an "A" in general physics along with a good MCAT Physical Sciences score than a lower grade in a calculus-based physics course. What's more, the Medical College Admission Test (MCAT), in its Physical Sciences subsection, tests NON-CALCULUS BASED PHYSICS. Remember, getting an "A" in general non-calculus based physics is hard enough and challenging anyway!

The same advice goes for courses in organic chemistry. If you have received a "C" in introductory organic chemistry and are not a chemistry major, you probably shouldn't try to "impress" a medical school admissions committee by taking a more advanced organic chemistry course. Do not let your "personal and academic" egos get in the way—trying to show that you "really do know organic chemistry" may just end your premed career. The proper place to prove your real knowledge will be on the MCAT—save it for then, and don't risk a low grade in the advanced course.

Keep in mind that you should avoid "academic double whammies"—situations where your GPA gets knocked down twice because you wrongfully chose the second course even with evidence of a "subpar" performance on the first introductory science or math course.

Remember, do not let your ego get in the way—you need to do what is RIGHT FOR YOU! "Staying within yourself" involves this and more—knowing your strengths and weaknesses so that you do not prematurely curtail your premed career. . . . Remember that "premedicine is not medicine" (see point number "Eight" in this chapter).

2. There is Really No Such Thing as "Majoring in Premed."

Remember that premedical courses are only a group of pre-selected courses used to evaluate candidates for medical school admission. The "basic four" (general chemistry/introductory biology/organic chemistry/introductory physics) are those courses that are also tested on the MCAT and are required by a vast majority of medical schools. (Calculus is also required or "recommended" by many schools but is not tested on the MCAT.)

3. Majoring in a Biological Science (*e.g.* Biology, Zoology, Microbiology, etc.) or A Physical Science (Chemistry Or Physics) is Not a Necessary Prerequisite for Getting Into Medical School.
This concept is discussed in detail in Chapter 8, "Selecting a Major."

4. You Can Major in Almost Any Subject When Applying to Medical School (Also See Chapter 8, "Selecting a Major").

For the most part, medical schools only require you to take the "basic four" premed science courses—general chemistry, introductory physics, organic chemistry, and introductory biology. Other courses, such as calculus and English will be required by some but "highly recommended" by most schools.

You should avoid, however, those majors on your campus that have the reputation of being the "easiest." Medical schools have vast experience working with undergraduate institutions and are fully aware of their academic majors/curricula.

5. Avoid Becoming Your School's Negative Symbol/Embodiment of "Mr./Ms. Premed."

During college, most premedical students usually show some of the negative signs and symptoms of "being" premed, but the real danger occurs if you "come down with the full blown disease." This principle is discussed further in Chapter 6, "Signs and Symptoms of Being Premed: Accentuating the Positive and Avoiding the Negative."

6. Going to a Highly Competitive College or University Will Not Necessarily Guarantee Admission Into Medical School.

The more important word here is "succeeding" (not just "going to one of these schools") at such a school. A school's reputation alone will never get you into medical school—it is the individual's overall achievements at such a school that will make the student a highly competitive applicant.

7. If Given The Chance, Take Every Early Opportunity To "Jump Start" Your Premedical Career By Taking A Good Foundation Of Science And Math Courses In High School.

Premedical students come from a large variety of academic backgrounds. In terms of preparation, some college freshmen come with minimal science backgrounds while others will have taken calculus courses along with "college level" chemistry, biology, and/or physics. If your high school offers "honors" or Advance Placement (AP) courses in some of the basic premedical sciences (chemistry, biology, physics), it would be advisable to take some/all of these courses; not only will you build an exceptional knowledge base, you will also develop the strong study skills necessary to excel in college. One key course (if offered) to take in high school is calculus. Understanding the material and doing well in that course will give you a head-start in college; not only should it help you to become more efficient with your study time, it will also be a great confidence booster. In a college calculus class, there will be many students who have never had calculus. They will need to spend extra time in this course because the material is entirely new to them. Many of these other students will also be premed and may be taking general chemistry and/or introductory biology. As you can see, taking some of those premed classes along with other courses can make freshman year quite challenging from the start. Having a good background in calculus, for example, will allow you to spend extra time with your remaining classes (You cannot, of course, "slack off" with your present calculus class). If you study hard, having a good science and/or math background will help you to master your course material, become more efficient with your time, and land you those top grades.

8. Premedicine Is Not Medicine.

To many premedical students, this may seem like a simple, obvious statement. Some students believe that if "I can take all the science and math that I can, medical school admission will be readily attainable." Why do the majority of premed students still major in a biological based science or a physical science (e.g. chemistry or physics)? . . . Because of the "absolute" belief that if they can survive the "rough and tumble" world of biology/premed, they will certainly gain admission into medical school and retain the "competitive edge" to both do well in med school and beyond. To really understand this premise (Premedicine is not medicine) is to truly "burst the premed bubble"—to realize that majoring in science IS NOT AN ABSOLUTE PREREQUISITE FOR MEDICAL SCHOOL ADMISSION. The bottom line is that "taking all the science you can" while an undergraduate may not make a big difference once you get to medical school; what will make the difference is if you SELECTIVELY take those courses that will INDEED MAKE A DIFFERENCE. There are really only a couple of courses on the undergraduate level that will ABSOLUTELY help you while in medical school and give you an ADVANTAGE DURING YOUR FIRST YEAR OF MEDICAL SCHOOL. These courses—PHYSIOLOGY and BIOCHEMISTRY—will only help you in medical school if: 1) you do not take the "watered-down," easier versions of these courses and 2) you work to "master the material" as if you were already in medical school.

The really good news for all students is that non-science majors who are fulfilling premedical requirements can take these same courses. Remember, you should major in an AREA THAT GENUINELY INTERESTS YOU. If that is in a biological science area then go for it! If you are a non-science major, you will still be able to schedule courses (physiology, biochemistry, histology, embryology, etc.) that will help you during your first year of medical school.

9. Strive to Get as Good of a Broad-Based Undergraduate Education as You Can.

If you follow this principle, you will avoid the mistakes made by thousands of medical students over the years who wished they could "go back and redo" their undergraduate course selections and/or major. Go to any medical school and you will more than likely hear students lamenting about their academic course selections as undergraduates. Most of the conversations you would hear usually begin in a similar manner: "I know hindsight is always 20/20, but too bad I wasn't in college now because I would have majored in another area"; "I wish I would have taken this course(s)" or "I wish I would not have taken this course(s)"; "When I had the opportunity in college, I really should have taken. . . ."

All of these statements can usually be heard during the first two years of medical school when basic medical sciences (such as anatomy, physiology, biochemistry, histology, pathology, microbiology, pharmacology, etc.) will be "crammed down your throat" six to eight hours per day. That is only in class time; the additional hours that are spent studying the material will seem almost endless. . . . The fact is that learning so much basic science during those first two years will make many students even "forget" that they are in medical school. . . . They may feel like Ph.D. students who are studying that particular subject (*e.g.* anatomy, biochemistry, physiology, etc.) as their major. It is, especially during these times of intensive study, when one becomes so focused on SCIENCE . . . SCIENCE . . . SCIENCE . . . that the previous lamentations about "what one should have studied" in undergraduate school are heard.

It is during these first two years that students truly discover that "science will be their life now and in their future." It will become difficult to become the well-rounded individuals they thought they would be as time, opportunity, and financial constraints become increasingly apparent. The easiest way to become that well-rounded physician you will want to be is to lay the groundwork in your undergraduate years. You can avoid these mistakes (the ones made by those lamenters who begrudgingly believe that they may have become too narrow-minded) by following some basic principles:

1. FOLLOW YOUR INTERESTS. . . . Follow your heart and your head when it comes to choosing your major. If you are a non-science major who is also premed, you have already developed a good game plan for becoming a well-rounded, broad-based, knowledgeable person.

2. If you are a science major and desire to take more non-science courses that interest you, do not hesitate to do it. Nowadays, almost all colleges have core course/liberal arts requirements that all students must fulfill. It might be a good idea to take those courses that both interest you and will be of benefit to you. Sometimes you may be tempted to take an easier course, but you must decide what a COLLEGE EDUCATION REALLY MEANS TO YOU! You should also carefully choose your electives. As your junior and senior years approach, you will have a "better feel for your schedule" and you will be able to plan your elective schedule. There may even be some semesters (especially in your senior year) that may allow room for two elective courses. If an "elective-of- interest" is only offered during one academic

semester, you should "look ahead" and plan an appropriate schedule. Remember, your senior year will be your last chance to take some of those courses that you "always wanted to take"—once medical school starts, there is no looking back.

10. <u>There Are Some Science Courses That You Should Take as an Undergraduate Which Will Help You Academically in Medical School.</u>

The "top priority" courses are PHYSIOLOGY and BIOCHEMISTRY. This principle is discussed further in Chapter 8, "Selecting a Major".

3
Qualities and Study Skills of Highly Efficient and Successful Students

Attaining very good grades at the college level, along with scoring well on standardized tests, appears to be the most important objective criteria in the medical school admissions application process. These two factors can help you get the most important interview in your early medical professional life. Getting those good grades and acceptable MCAT scores will really be the culmination of study techniques and highly effective personal habits, many of which were developed even before one's college years. For other premedical students, the self-discovery process of knowing "what it takes" to become successful took longer; but the end results are the same. Receiving that medical school acceptance letter provides the proof that these students have "all the right academic stuff" to succeed in the rigors of professional school.

The bottom line is that it is never too late to become a highly efficient and successful student. You don't have to be the valedictorian or salutatorian of your high school class to go to medical school someday; you don't even have to be in the top ten percent of your high school class. There are many students who "awake academically in college"; this is usually a reflection of a student finding an academic area of interest which truly interests and motivates him/her. At the same time, however, a highly competitive job and career market has transformed some "would-be slackers" into "doers." Obviously, if you have done extremely well in high school, you cannot rest on those laurels. College, especially premedicine, is a brand new ballgame; those who make it through the "premed rigors" are all intelligent, highly motivated, and goal-oriented individuals.

At every new level of your academic career, there will be more that is expected from you . . . . Premedical studies are more difficult than those in high school . . . . Admission into medical school is much more competitive than getting into a college . . . . The volume of med school material to be learned will make the content of an organic chemistry class appear "extremely manageable"! . . . During your residency and professional career, there will be numerous demands on your time and personal life . . . . What's more, there will always be standardized tests to take . . . . Medical licensing boards (three separate tests), residency exams, specialty tests, sub-specialty boards, re-certification exams . . . . Well, I think you've gotten the picture!

The positive personal qualities and study skills that you develop early in your academic career will enhance your ability to succeed along every step of the physician pathway. This chapter provides numerous "pearls of advice" to help you succeed in reaching your potential as a premedical student. While some of these techniques may seem obvious to you as a student, others will certainly not be. One great advantage of learning about these techniques is that you will be able to use some of them in both medical school and later in your professional life. Another advantage of being introduced to a variety of very practical skills and qualities is that you will be able to develop your own "individualized secrets to success." Though there are "no 100 percent guarantees in life" (a cliché that is especially applicable in today's volatile job and career market), there are ways to reach your potential and enhance your chances of medical school admission.

Before discussing each one in detail, I have provided the list of subject topics that are covered in this chapter. This will allow you to use the listing as a quick reference guide when applying the appropriate principles to your own academic and personal life.

List of Topics

1. Study to succeed.

2. Know what is expected of you in your courses.

3. Get to know your professors/instructors/teaching assistants.

4. "Actively use" your textbooks/manuals/handouts and other course materials.

5. Use old exams when you study.

6. Don't overextend your academic science course load.

7. Studying by yourself vs. a study group.

8. Make sure your surroundings are conducive for effective study.

9. Realize the "study content" of each course so that you can use the appropriate study strategies and methods for success.

10. Take the INITIATIVE and seek help in your coursework.

11. Don't underestimate the value of commercial solution manuals, review books, and summary guides.

12. Be well organized, know how to manage your time, and don't procrastinate.

13. Be attentive to course details.

14. Know how to be a "stress buster".

15. Keep a balanced lifestyle.

1. STUDY TO SUCCEED.

While this point may seem obvious to the reader, its basic tenets are not practiced by all students. "Studying to succeed" is a "frame of mind," an "attitude", a belief that doing your academic work "half-way" is just not good enough. It is this frame of mind that helps one's "discipline shine through." It allows you to realize what has to take precedence; if that means studying the weekend for that organic chemistry exam on Monday, so be it; you will probably have the next couple of weekends to balance out your personal and social life. Even when you're stuck in the library on those weekends, it shouldn't be for the entire weekend. The law of diminishing returns elucidates the point that you cannot study too many hours straight—you have to realize "when" and "how" to take breaks in order to revive yourself for the next "round of study hours." "All study with no breaks" will make you a "dull premedical student" and will help exacerbate those negative premedical symptoms discussed in Chapter 6, "Signs and Symptoms of Being Premed: Accentuating the Positive and Avoiding the Negative."

It is often difficult to figure out why some students (including both successful and unsuccessful premed students) choose to "just get through" a course, a lab, or an assigned research paper. Why do some students spend all those countless hours in lab yet not put in the proper effort when writing the lab report? Why not spend those extra few hours perfecting that term paper? . . . It may make the difference between getting an "A" or a "B" or a "B" or a "C." Realistically, you cannot expect to get an "A" all of the time. (The myth of medical schools filling up their classes with 4.00 students having perfect MCAT scores is just that . . . a myth.) What you really have to look at is the following: did I put the proper EFFORT into this test or assignment?

There are, of course, factors that may be totally out of your control. For example, the test may have been so ridiculously difficult that very few people did well on it. The bottom line is that you should look at YOURSELF and ask: "No matter what the grade is, do I give myself an "A," "B," or "C" for MY EFFORT"? Whatever your "personal grade" is on your efforts, YOU MUST AVOID THE COMMON MISTAKE OF BEING TOO HARD ON YOURSELF. You must provide your own positive reinforcement: "Whatever happened on this test or assignment I can ACTIVELY learn from the experience and improve the outcome for the next time." You should also never be afraid to say "I don't know." This realization will help motivate you to become a better student and to seek outside help as needed. The phrase "knowledge is not knowing everything but knowing where to find it" really is TRUE; this will become particularly evident in medical school.

2.   KNOW WHAT IS EXPECTED OF YOU IN YOUR COURSES.

At the start of each semester, list the date/due date of each major exam/quiz/lab report/essay/research paper and the approximate percentage each is worth towards the final grade; keeping yourself organized in this manner will prevent any "undue surprises" and anxiety caused by the fact that you suddenly have five assignments/tests/reports due in one week. You will undoubtedly have to face an academic onslaught of assignments throughout your academic career; if you are prepared, however, there should be no sudden surprises. Knowing the course expectations ahead of time should help you adequately PREPARE and BUDGET YOUR TIME.

3.   GET TO KNOW YOUR PROFESSORS/INSTRUCTORS/TEACHING ASSISTANTS.

In very large courses, some students simply remain a "number" and not a "name." (If a student does not take the initiative, the same thing can also occur in a course with a small enrollment!) Professors even complain sometimes that office hours are held with relatively few or no students coming to ask about lectures or problem sets. Remember, you are investing time, energy, and tuition into your college learning experience; you need to take advantage of every learning opportunity that is available. If you don't understand certain concepts or are having difficulty solving various science or math problems, take the INITIATIVE and see your instructor(s). Allowing the course content "to get away from you" can prove disastrous at exam time. If you let all the problems you don't understand or can't solve pile up to the end, you will cheat yourself out of both a rewarding learning experience and an opportunity to earn a higher grade. Getting to know your professors will also help you when you need a letter of recommendation for medical school. If your instructor gets to know about your personal qualities, you can be sure that a letter of recommendation will more than just discuss your "A" in general chemistry. Also, don't hesitate to seek a professor's advice about a summer internship or job, especially if it relates to an area of interest he/she has discussed or researched. (At times, the ones who know you best—parents/professors/counselors—can provide constructive input when deciding about a summer work opportunity.)

It is also important to be "yourself" around your professor. The exhibition of negative "premed symptoms" (such as "over-aggressiveness" or being "artificially nice") does not bode well when it comes time for a letter of recommendation.

4. "ACTIVELY USE" YOUR TEXTBOOKS/MANUALS/HANDOUTS AND OTHER COURSE MATERIALS.

Well, you may ask . . . What does THAT mean? Simply put, don't hesitate to underline, highlight text, write notes in your margins, or paper clip notes into your textbooks and other class materials; every time you read and review your materials, the salient points from that chapter will be better remembered. (Some students take a "hands off" approach when it comes to their books—they want them to look like new at the end of the semester or school year so that they can get a good trade-in-value. Remember, resale values on your textbooks won't fulfill most students expectations. Second, editions change every several years, so there's a chance that your book will not be re-sold.)

If you have old exams available from that course, make notational marks in your book on particular concepts or problem types that were previously tested. Every test in the basic premedical sciences usually has questions or problems that separate the "A"s from the "B"s; in some instances, some questions can be so difficult or esoteric that very few students answer them correctly. Make special notations in your books and other class materials on exactly these DIFFICULT POINTS; you will see that it will MAKE A DIFFERENCE.

When it comes to your basic science textbooks (Biology/General Chemistry/Physics/Organic Chemistry), it is my opinion that you should keep them as references when studying for the MCAT. The key word is "REFERENCE"; with all the top-notch MCAT preparation books and courses, it would be very inefficient to read and study your textbooks cover to cover when studying for the MCAT. What you should do is use your textbooks, class notes, and completed problem sets as complete reference guides to questions and problems you don't understand in your MCAT study/review materials.

Commercial MCAT prep courses and books usually have fair to excellent summaries of all the four basic sciences which are tested. If you don't fully understand the summary or need more detailed explanation of a particular topic, you can then use your school course materials and textbooks as a reference source.

5. USE OLD EXAMS WHEN YOU STUDY.

The content of your coursework can be presented in only a finite number of ways. This same thing can be said of the exams you will take in your courses. Similar problems or concepts (and even sometimes the identical questions are asked) that are on old exams will usually reappear on your present exam. You will also get a good grasp of the instructors' testing methods (FAMILIARITY PRODUCES EFFICIENCY): problem sets, true/false, multiple choice, "multiple/multiple" choice questions (where one or more answers can be correct), essays, short answer, "matching", fill-in-the-blank questions, etc. Instructors have favorite ways of testing, and old exams are key to understanding their methods.

Knowing an instructor's method(s) of testing should not be taken lightly. You may know how to solve every quantitative problem in your chemistry text, but you may walk into class and see that half of the exam consists of essay questions. You need to be prepared for your instructor's type of exam. . . . There should be no real surprises when it comes to testing methodology. Professors usually inform their students before the exam about the different sections (true/false, problems, multiple choice, etc.) on the exam. Having old exams should take the "mystery out of trick questions" and will help you understand the mechanics of writing a good essay or short answer.

When using old exams, there are a few pearls of advice worth noting. First, the use of old exams should serve only as "study aides" and should never be used as a substitute for the course. I knew a small group of students who usually crammed the night before a general chemistry exam and used old exams as their only source for studying. They consistently received "C"s (and even some "D"s) and never learned that ACTIVE STUDYING meant more than just putting in an effort studying old exams. These students dropped their medical school aspirations within a year and left science coursework altogether. Second, many successful students start looking at old exams after they have thoroughly studied and reviewed the course material for the test. The review of old exams usually begins any time from several days to the night before the exam. This technique has proven to be successful as long as the course material has already been thoroughly studied and mastered. It is also assumed that all the problem sets and assignments have been worked out and completely understood.

To make your studying even more efficient, I suggest that you start looking at the old exams right from the start for those chapters/topics that are to be tested. Realizing what you will need to know ahead of time will make your study plan even more effective. The most successful study habits assume that the student will learn and master all the material that will appear on an exam. That material will probably consist of textbook content/problem sets/lectures/labs and notes from review sessions. Mastering the course content and thoroughly knowing every old exam is an unbeatable combination when test time comes along! Mastering the material in this manner will help you get those exam questions that always make the difference between an "A" and a "B." Going through the material repeatedly and with a thorough understanding of it, will usually translate into both an "A" grade and a personal satisfaction of academic achievement.

6. DON'T OVEREXTEND YOUR ACADEMIC SCIENCE COURSE LOAD.

The time to overextend your science course load will be in medical school . . . NOT NOW (In medical school you will not have a choice.) . . . . At the present time enjoy your college experience. There is no advantage of taking too many science courses every semester ("all the science I can take" approach). Don't let your ego get in the way . . . .

If it does, you risk poor grades and high anxiety states.

"Staying within yourself" again repeats itself as a major theme in achieving success as a premedical student. If you take an "appropriate schedule" for yourself, you will have more time to concentrate on the subject matter, really "learn" the material, and maintain excellent grades. You will also lessen the "stress level" in your life by creating a reasonable schedule that will allow more time for extracurricular activities and a social life.

7.   STUDYING BY YOURSELF VS. A STUDY GROUP.

Depending on the course material and what you want to accomplish, there is a place for a GOOD, DISCIPLINED STUDY GROUP. For the most part, you should study alone. You can usually get more done, review the material several times, and more easily avoid distraction. A study group, if organized to achieve the APPROPRIATE GOALS, can serve as an excellent ADJUNCT to your individualized study sessions. Study groups can prove to be quite effective if they are small (2-4 students; some even consider (4) people too large for a study group.) and consist of DISCIPLINED, COOPERATIVE, and RELIABLE students. If you put together such a group (even yourself and one other student), make sure each student realizes the goals to be achieved. Science courses which have numerous quantitative problems to solve can be conducive to this type of study session. For example, general chemistry and introductory physics usually have so many problems at the end of each chapter that it would be difficult for one person to do every one of them. Even instructors realize this and assign only the "even" or "odd" numbered problems at the end of the chapter. (For exam purposes, however, the whole chapter is "fair game" and that includes the content of all the problems). The best way to really understand courses such as these is TO DO ALL OF THE PROBLEMS. (That is where your reliable and disciplined study group partner(s) can make the difference.) I personally used this method (I had one study partner and we did ALL of the problems) for general chemistry and physics, and the academic dividends paid handsomely; besides "thoroughly acing" these courses, I felt I had a very THOROUGH UNDERSTANDING of the material even before I started preparing for the MCAT. Total familiarity with problem solving techniques will make your MCAT studying even more efficient. . . . You should be able to say, "I've seen that material before, I KNOW that material and now I have to master it for the most important test of my young professional life." Remember, FAMILIARITY and REPETITION pay off in the end. . . . STUDYING TO SUCCEED is more than "just putting in the hours"; it is a "frame of mind," an "academic attitude" that will carry you to success.

When using the study group approach, each student must know their assignments and deadlines. The work should be shared equally and complete solutions should be written in sufficient detail for each student to understand the "thought processes" in solving the problems. Obviously, as a courtesy to your other group member(s), you should also photocopy your solutions so that everyone has a "study copy." It is also important to keep in communication with each other about individual progress with the problem sets. There will always be some very difficult problems that may need special insight. If you cannot solve a certain problem(s), then perhaps your study partner can (You can then "trade" some problems so that all the work is shared appropriately.); you should, however, make every attempt to solve the difficult problems. . . . You can always seek help from a professor, teaching assistant, or fellow student. . . . Don't be timid; take the initiative! There are also many commercial books on the market that have "working solutions" ("step-by-step" solutions) to almost every type of problem. These books usually provide that extra insight to help you solve those difficult math, chemistry, or physics problems. You will see that with a successful and efficient study group, you will have access to the solutions of hundreds of problems you probably would never have time to do yourself.

Lastly, avoid the pitfalls that make study groups break up. The common themes of procrastination, "not sharing the work" and not meeting the deadlines, have caused many study groups to become dysfunctional (Don't let this happen to yours!). Always keep your group's goals in mind: Not only do you want to obtain good grades, but you want to MASTER and UNDERSTAND the material.

8. MAKE SURE YOUR SURROUNDINGS ARE CONDUCIVE FOR EFFECTIVE STUDY.

Establish some favorite, QUIET study spots for yourself. . . . undergraduate libraries, classrooms, study hall areas, empty offices, your room (when the dorm or apartment is quiet), or even the medical school library ("I study here. . . . Someday I'll be here!). Don't study with a TV, radio, or stereo on; how many times have you been in the library near someone who puts on a cassette player with headphones? You know what I'm talking about. . . . It's an absolute nuisance!

Some students believe they can study with any type of noise around them; this is just NOT TRUE. Even over a short period of time your concentration abilities become diminished both consciously and subconsciously. Study time really does become less efficient and this ultimately translates into lower grades. Try studying like this in medical school, and you won't get very far.

There are also other small pearls of advice which can help you enhance your study environment. While studying, you should avoid laying around too long on a comfortable chair or couch. If you do this consistently, you may find that sleep time may outdistance study time. Second, don't eat big meals before you study or take a test. (Remember, you need to feed your brain and not overfeed your stomach!) You also need to take effective study breaks. That may mean taking a short ten-minute walk, sitting back in a chair with your eyes closed for a few minutes, or telephoning a friend. You need to do those things for yourself which will help break up the intensity of your study sessions.

Libraries and designated study areas are usually filled with study cubicles—desks/tables which have wooden dividers on three sides. Avoid sitting at this type of a desk for too long of a time. Sitting in an "open" and "airy" environment where you can look out a window or easily glance at distant objects helps the student feel "less enclosed." Studying at an open desk or table also allows you the space to spread out all of your study materials and have easier access to them.

It is also a very good idea to change your study environment. Always studying in the same desk in the same building can force you into a "study rut." By all means, AVOID THIS; you would be surprised how many different places on campus you can find if you just take the INITIATIVE. If there are graduate or professional schools (law, medical, dental, etc.) on campus, you should consider using their libraries to study. These libraries tend to be very quiet and are open longer than the undergraduate ones.

9. REALIZE THE "STUDY CONTENT" OF EACH COURSE SO THAT YOU USE THE APPROPRIATE STUDY STRATEGIES AND METHODS FOR SUCCESS.

You will be expected to understand general concepts, theories, and principles in all of your courses (whether it be a natural science, humanities, or social science course). Success in some of your courses will rely on the rote memorization of voluminous facts (*e.g.* biology, organic chemistry). Other disciplines, such as general chemistry, general physics, and calculus, will need the student to completely master quantitative problem solving techniques. (Solving hundreds of problems in these areas will give you the mental discipline to think like a "chemist" or a "physicist." This discipline pays off when these areas are tested on the MCAT.)

Success in other areas such as the humanities (*e.g.* English and American literature, comparative literature) and the social sciences (*e.g.* history, economics, political science, sociology, etc.) will depend on both your reading comprehension and communication skills. You will have to become an "analytical and critical thinker" in these areas and be able to write informative, logical, and well-written essays. These other disciplines may also use the traditional techniques of testing (true/false, multiple choice, etc.), so you need to know your instructors' methods for the exam.

10. TAKE THE INITIATIVE AND SEEK HELP IN YOUR COURSEWORK.

You have to know when and how to seek help . . . and the earlier the better! You will have access to numerous outlets for "first-aid" in the "ailing aspects" of your coursework: professors, teaching assistants, lab instructors, study groups, review sessions, other students, tutoring services (paid and volunteer), commercial reference and review books, etc. The list of such opportunities should be optimistically reassuring to the student. . . .

Help is there if you seek it!

11. DON'T UNDERESTIMATE THE VALUE OF COMMERCIAL SOLUTION MANUALS, REVIEW BOOKS, AND SUMMARY GUIDES.

These books should not replace your textbooks, notes, and other class materials but should serve as supplements in helping you do well in your coursework. At the end of this chapter, I have listed a number of these references that are popular with both high school and college students. (These are not sponsored endorsements of these books; I am not getting paid for listing them in my book.)

12. BE WELL ORGANIZED, KNOW HOW TO MANAGE YOUR TIME, AND DON'T PROCRASTINATE.

(Obviously, these statements are easier said than done. . . .   They will, however, remain the key concepts for your success now, in medical school, and during your professional life.)

There is a variety of methods which students use to achieve these goals: "To do" lists, calendars, detailed assignment booklets, "reminder" notes, etc. The general rule is that you must use a system that WORKS FOR YOU! As an undergraduate, your studies should remain the number one priority, but there will always be other responsibilities that will force you to do a "balancing act": family matters, extracurricular activities, part-time jobs, personal matters, etc. . . .   These will all compete for your time. The earlier you learn organizational and time-management skills, the earlier you will both realize success and maintain it at an acceptable level.

KNOWING your priorities ("school is number one") can help you avoid both academic and emotional crises: "all-nighters", anxiety, panic. . . .   All of these are negative factors that will ultimately diminish your performance. . . .   POOR PREPARATION ALWAYS EQUATES WITH POOR PERFORMANCE. Putting off doing those general chemistry problem sets will only mean cramming at the end. . . .   An overly anxious mind tends not to be very receptive to concentrating and learning large amounts of material. Even if that "study style" ("procrastination") works for you as an undergraduate, it will not work for you in medical school.

13. BE ATTENTIVE TO COURSE DETAILS.

Knowing the details of your course material can help make the difference between an "A" and a "B"; it can also be a key factor in making you one of the top students in the course (It is also excellent preparation for medical school). Subject areas that sometimes seem too difficult to understand or would make "trivia questions" usually appear on exams. Even topics that professors seemed to "skim over" in class pop up again on examinations.

"Seeing the forest for the trees" has always seemed to be a guiding principle when it comes to analyzing and studying course concepts and principles; you will hear this many times throughout your academic career; but the truth is you really have to "know the trees" (all of the details) in order to understand the forest. Let's face it. . . . Just knowing and understanding concepts will get you in the ballpark. . . . But everyone really wants to hit the home run. . . . Well then, you have to know the course DETAILS. This will be good practice for medical school where professors always seem to test the "trivial" and "obscure" details of your course materials. Medical students and physicians alike would agree that just knowing the "concepts" for a medical school exam will not be "good enough"; basically you need to know "everything" for your medical school exams.

As undergraduates, you must first obtain an excellent conceptual understanding of your course materials. Once you obtain this comprehensive understanding, you then need to learn and memorize the remaining details. Don't be afraid to be very attentive to these details—it will make you a top student on your exams, and you'll be well prepared for the testing techniques utilized in medical school.

14. KNOW HOW TO BE A "STRESS BUSTER."

When the going gets tough. . . . It's time to help relax your mind. At times, your life will inevitably seem out of balance ("so much to do in so little time"). Remember that exams, lab reports, and research paper deadlines are a "way of life." Remember that these stressful times (when it seems that "everything is due") do not last forever. . . . They will pass. . . . But it will be your coping mechanisms (organizational and time-management skills, avoiding procrastination) that will help you be a successful premed student. Getting adequate sleep, food, and exercise will be important factors in counteracting all of those potential stressful academic situations.

Eating a good "non-indulging" breakfast the morning of an exam will help increase your performance levels. Cereal, juice, oatmeal, and fruit are all examples of foods that are light on the stomach but highly nutritious for the soon to be "exam tested brain."

Even when you're on a study marathon, do something that will ease the tension—take a walk or a run, do some calisthenics, flip on the TV for a few minutes, play your musical instrument, talk to a good friend, call home. . . .   All of these, along with many other methods, DO WORK! Find methods that work for you and practice them. Remember to TAKE THE TIME to be your own "STRESS BUSTER."

Another method that works for many students (especially around final exam time) relates both positive thinking with delayed gratification. "Positive imaging" takes only a few minutes but helps break up long study hours and helps ease the tension that you may be feeling both emotionally and physically. You need to think for a few minutes (not daydream for hours) of the activities you enjoy the most: going out with your best friends, playing basketball, hiking in the woods, playing the piano, watching a beautiful sunset, etc.; once the semester is over, you should do some of your favorite activities; but while you're going through the "tough academic times," use them as "positive imaging"—a reward to be enjoyed in the very near future. You will undoubtedly see that when you partake in these activities after the semester, you will have an even better appreciation of them!

15. KEEP A BALANCED LIFESTYLE.

Your social life, extracurricular activities, sports, volunteer work, part-time student employment, musical interests, family life, and hobbies are all important factors in making YOU WHO YOU ARE. Keep participating in those constructive activities, but do it in a "balanced way." Again, the principles of time management, organizational skills, and delayed gratification should help you reach that goal of a balanced lifestyle.

Examples of Commercial Review Books, Summary Guides, and Solution Manuals

Many of these books are excellent; they not only discuss every concept and principle relevant to your course but also provide the details that are necessary to master your coursework. Included in these series of books are manuals that have solutions to almost every imaginable quantitative problem or question in those science and math courses (calculus/ general chemistry/organic chemistry/physics) that seem most challenging to the premedical student. One important "pearl of advice" when buying these books is to CHOOSE CAREFULLY—choose the books that will probably work best for you. Remember, these books are course supplements and not substitutes! (NOTE: The topics that are listed are in the science and math areas. Some of these book series also have resources for other topics in the social and behavioral sciences and humanities.)

1. Barron's *The Easy Way Series* (Barron's Educational Series, Inc.).
   (*e.g. Chemistry the Easy Way*)

Subject Topic Examples:

- Anatomy and Physiology
- Biology
- Calculus
- Chemistry
- Mathematics
- Physics

2. Barron's *EZ-101 Study Keys*.

Subject Topic Examples:

- Biology
- Chemistry
- Physics

3. Cliffs *Quick Review* (Cliffs Notes, Inc.)

Subject Topic Examples:

- Biology
- Calculus
- Chemistry
- Physics

4. Doubleday *Made Simple Books Series*. *(e.g. Chemistry Made Simple)*

Subject Topic Examples:

- Chemistry
- Intermediate Algebra and Analytic Geometry
- Physics

5. Harcourt Brace *College Outline Series*.

Subject Topic Examples:

- Calculus
- College Algebra
- College Chemistry
- College Physics
- Geometry
- Trigonometry
- University Physics I
- University Physics II

6. HarperCollins *College Outline Series*.

Subject Topic Examples:

- Chemistry
- Organic Chemistry
- Calculus

7. Bob Muller's books (McGraw-Hill Companies, Inc.).

- *PreCalculus Helper*
- *Calculus I Helper*
- *Calculus II Helper*

8. Research and Education Association's (REA) *Problem Solvers*.

Subject Topic Examples:

- Advanced Calculus
- Algebra and Trigonometry
- Calculus
- Chemistry
- Biology
- Genetics
- Physics
- Mathematics for Engineers
- Organic Chemistry
- Physics
- Pre-Calculus
- Physical Chemistry

9. Research and Education Association's (REA):

- *Verbal Builder for Admission and Standardized Tests*
- *Math Builder for Admission and Standardized Tests*
- *Achievement Tests: SAT II and Subject Tests*

10. Research and Education Association's (REA) *The High School Tutor Series.*

Subject Topic Examples:

- Algebra
- Biology
- Chemistry
- Earth Science
- Geometry
- Physics
- Pre-Calculus
- SAT I Math
- SAT I Verbal
- Probability
- Trigonometry

11. Schaum's *Solved Problems* series (McGraw-Hill Companies, Inc.). 3000 solved problems in each of the following areas:

- Biology
- Calculus
- Chemistry
- Chemistry
- Organic Chemistry
- Physics

12. Schaum's *Outlines* (McGraw-Hill Companies, Inc.).

Subject Topic Examples:

- Calculus
- Physics

Biology Areas
- Biology
- Human Anatomy and Physiology
- Molecular and Cell Biology
- Zoology

Chemistry Areas
- Biochemistry
- College Chemistry
- Organic Chemistry

4

Being Premed and Choosing
Your Undergraduate School:
An Introduction

Whether you are age 18, 28, or 38, choosing to become premed (and STICKING WITH IT!) will be one of the MAJOR decisions in your life. Making your college or university choice will have a direct effect on your life as a premed for the next two, three, or four years (depending on where you are in your academic program: college freshman or college grad fulfilling medical school requirements). The next chapter discusses in detail the "nuts and bolts" of choosing your college. Before reading that chapter, there are a couple of issues that must be considered in order to make yourself a well informed college applicant who "also happens to be premed."

The first issue is a question that must be addressed up front—"What is the acceptance rate for medical school applicants for that school?" (a/k/a: Does that college have high success rates in getting its students into medical school?) Is the acceptance rate greater or less than 50 percent . . . 70 percent . . . 80 percent . . . or greater than 90 percent? It is obvious that the higher the percentage, the better opportunity you will have of getting accepted into medical school.

Keeping this in mind, please be aware of potentially ambiguous statements issued by colleges/advisory or career offices in their brochures, pamphlets, or catalogs about their premedical program. At times, you really need "JUST THE RIGHT FACTS." (Sometimes nothing may be in print, but you will hear statements from premed and career advisors about their high medical school acceptance rates. At the same time, however, colleges also desire the "increased prestige" of boasting about their "impeccable premed reputation" and their "outstanding record of medical school acceptances.") Today, many colleges are competing for a declining population base of college-age applicants (compared to the 1960s-1980s) and find it financially necessary to market their strengths and academic highpoints.

These ambiguous promotional statements can sometimes be viewed as "badly written prose," "marketing ploys," or "innocent mistakes." Remember that some of these statements

---

can appear misleading to the "unwary eye and ear" of an eager prospective premed student. To help yourself through this "mystifying maze," make sure you truly understand what is being told to you. There are a variety of potentially ambiguous statements that could mislead an aspiring premedical student. The following statements serve as examples of what to "look out for" (Interpretations of these statements follow in the next section):

1. Our premed students' average GPA for medical school admission is 3.6.

2. "Over 85 percent of our premedical students get admitted to medical school."

3. We typically have an acceptance rate of approximately 80 percent.

4. If you have a 3.75 from our school, there's over a 90 percent chance of being admitted into medical school.

5. Over 95 percent of our applicants get admitted to a health professional school.

Please be aware of the "words and phrases" that are sometimes used in these statements:

1.. "Average GPA" may not give the student the whole picture of the kind of grades needed from your undergraduate school. The type of information that can be even more useful is the GPA breakdowns (e.g. average/median; science GPA/overall GPA) of minority vs. non-minority applicants or science majors vs. non-science majors. The "median GPA" may give a more accurate description: "Half the students above, as well as half the students below this GPA, get into medical school." Besides GPA information, it will be important for the aspiring premedical college applicant to ask about the other key component for medical school admission: How do students from your college do on the MCATs (average scores, range of scores, what is the strongest subject(s) or the weakest one(s). . . . Why?).

2. "Admission into medical school." Believe it or not, even this term can be very misleading. Medical schools would include allopathic (M.D.), osteopathic (D.O.), and foreign medical schools. If you know, for example, that the college got ten students into foreign medical schools, six into D.O. schools but only two students into M.D. schools, you would probably consider another undergraduate institution. You need to know the acceptance rates and types of schools (e.g. M.D., D.O., and foreign) where students obtain admission.

3. Words like "typical," "average," or "approximate" again may be misleading when describing acceptance rates into medical school. The words, "typically 80 percent" or an "average of 80 percent" do no indicate recent trends or an exact admissions figure. For example, a school may have acceptance rates over the last five years of 90 percent/100 percent/90 percent/60 percent and 60 percent; as you can see, the average is 80 percent, but there is a

large downward trend in medical school acceptances! Unless the school can fully and adequately explain this discrepancy, you may not want to go there!

4. "If you have a 3.75 GPA from our school. . . ." The use of GPAs can again be very misleading. A GPA of 3.75 and above would, of course, describe a "top student" at any college or university. If an undergraduate school uses a GPA statistic, does that number include both types of majors (science and non-science majors) who fulfilled premed requirements? If all students with high GPAs did not get admitted into medical school, what explains these discrepancies (subpar MCAT scores, "bland" interviews, etc.)? One must also note that the vast majority of successful medical school applicants usually have GPAs ranging from 3.3 to 4.0.

    What are the success rates for these applicants at that particular college or university? (Remember, medical schools do not fill their classes with 4.0 students with extremely high MCAT scores.)

5. "Get admitted to a Health Professional School." This is the ULTIMATE MISLEADING STATEMENT to aspiring premeds and future M.D.'s. "Health professional school" can mean almost any type of program besides medical school—Podiatry (DPM), dentistry (DDS, DMD), chiropractic school (D.C.), Optometry (O.D.), Occupational or physical therapy (OT/PT), or even veterinarian school (DVM).

When explaining medical school admission rates, these categories should be kept separate: Medical school is medical school!; Podiatry school is podiatry school!; Dental school is for aspiring dentists!

One should also follow one additional "pearl of advice." During the college application process, try to get a feel for the number of freshmen premeds at your prospective schools. (Remember, any one can "declare themselves as premed," but the reasons for dropping the program can be numerous and varied.) For example, going to a college with 500 freshmen premeds may not be ideal for you if the "premed class" whittles down to 40 or 50 medical school applicants by senior year. (What's more, not all of these students may be admitted to medical school.) Some of these schools may be considered to be "highly competitive" with "stellar premed programs." You may be better off going to a school with both a good, established premed program ("a proven track record") but fewer premed students. "To be finished with premed" before you really even start it or "get into it" could be a professional tragedy. Remember, job satisfaction is usually a very high priority in most people's lives. No job is absolutely perfect, but LIKING WHAT YOU DO when you wake up every morning is not only one of life's greatest satisfactions, it is really a true gift. (The medical profession, when compared to other jobs, careers, and professions, has a very high rate of satisfaction.)

Again, the ultimate choice has to be yours. . . .   You need to be comfortable with your college choice while STAYING WITHIN YOURSELF. . . .   If you feel that you are well prepared academically for a "big time premed program" at a prestigious school, then you may have found your answer; this is not the answer, however, for many premed students who make the right college choice for themselves by looking at a number of factors (many of which will be addressed in the next chapter) to help answer the most important question—IS THIS COLLEGE RIGHT FOR ME?

Any college with a premed program should be able to address all the matters discussed in this chapter. There should be established statistics and records (especially recent statistics for that year and a few previous years) regarding their success at medical school admission. If an answer cannot be readily addressed, the resources should at least be available for the advisory office to give you a well-informed answer by a reasonable date. You should probably consider not attending that school if any of the following happen to you: 1) If you do not get satisfactory answers to your questions or if the premed advisory office is "too evasive" . . . 2) If the school's advisory office develops an "attitude" toward you as an applicant or considers you "too pushy" regarding your requests. (At the same time, the applicant's request/questions should also be "reasonable.").

Finally, in many cases, premedical advisors prepare an ongoing list of where students are accepted. You should ask the counseling office to see that information for the current year. There should also be a final listing of all medical school acceptances from the previous year that should also prove to be very helpful. Also, don't hesitate to get your parents involved in the "premedical inquiry process." You will see that WHEN PARENTS ASK QUESTIONS, COLLEGES DO LISTEN! (Colleges, after all, do know that most parents do pay/help pay the higher education bills!)

5

Choosing Your
College Or University

In choosing a college or university, many students take the advice of counselors, parents, friends, and family members: "Go to the best school in which you can gain admission." In today's world, outside pressures such as financial constraints may limit a student's college choice. This is especially true when the student has a long-term goal of attending a graduate or professional school. If you overextend yourself financially as an undergraduate, medical school may prove to be an uphill monetary struggle. There are, of course, ways to ease that burden: Attend a lower tuition medical school in your home state and/or join the military on one of their scholarship programs. (Keep in mind, however, that even some state schools are becoming very expensive; if you join the military, you will owe service time for each year of your scholarship.)

Whether or not you may need financial aid as an undergraduate or as a medical student, you still have to make that most fundamental choice: Is this college RIGHT FOR ME, and will it HELP ADVANCE MY CAREER GOALS?

Some premed students choose the undergraduate school that they believe will give them the best opportunity to gain admission into medical school. Remember, NO COLLEGE CAN GUARANTEE YOUR ADMISSION INTO MEDICAL SCHOOL. Some colleges might be able to increase your chances for admission, but the bottom line is that you must have the grades and the will to succeed. It is not your undergraduate school that will gain your admission to medical school—IT IS ONLY YOU—your grades, accomplishments, and personal qualities. It is a well-known fact that if you walk into all first-year medical school classes, you will discover a wide array of colleges and universities attended by those students. In terms of representation, there will be many state schools (with various branch campuses represented), small liberal arts colleges, and in some cases, schools that some people have never even heard about; at many medical schools, Ivy League and "Ivy-type" schools are in the definite minority when it comes to student body representation. No matter what the undergraduate institution is, however, the student in that medical school class seat will be well qualified and will have earned his/her right to be there.

In summary, there are three major principles that the aspiring premed college applicant should keep in mind: First, medical schools admit students from almost any accredited four-year undergraduate institution. Second, the type of ACADEMIC CREDENTIALS you present to the medical school admissions committee is more important than the TYPE of school you attended. (Of course, the combination of being a very successful student at a "top notch" undergraduate institution would increase your chances of admission. Remember, however, there are still no 100 percent guarantees!) Third, choosing an undergraduate school SOLELY as a "means to an end" (gaining medical school admission) may not be judicious. In making your college choice, you have to PICK THE SCHOOL that is RIGHT FOR YOU!

How Do You Know What School Is Right For You?

There are a variety of factors to consider when making the very important and most fundamental decision regarding a college choice. Your college years will serve as the building blocks for both your personal development and for your future career. These years will be a turning point in your life, a time in which you will grow from a high school teenager to a "real-life adult", accompanied by all of the responsibilities, duties, and benefits.

The numerous factors to consider when choosing a college can be divided in the following manner: academic curriculum and faculty; costs and financial aid; school's prestige and reputation; professional, graduate school, and job placement; pre-professional counseling and advisory services; extracurricular activities and social life; campus facilities and their accessibility; and other issues (transportation, safety, etc.). Though the following list of factors attempts to be "all-inclusive," there will always be (and should be) other questions asked by prospective college applicants. Obtaining answers to your additional questions may even make your college choice the right one for you! (Note: These lists in this chapter are only a short summary of factors to be considered. Their main goal is to help expand an aspiring premedical student's view of college choices. Remember, medical school admission does not rest solely on the name and reputation of your undergraduate institution. What's more, there are numerous guides and books on "how to choose a college," some of which are listed in the reference section after this chapter.)

Factors and Questions to Consider When Choosing
a College or University

1. ACADEMIC CURRICULUM AND FACULTY

    1. Can all the premedical requirements be met at that school?

    2. School's academic schedule: semester/trimester/quarter hours?

3. Strength of science and math departments.

4. Teacher/student ratio (undergraduate).

5. Can I "double major"? What combinations are possible?

6. Does the school have the major(s) that I am considering? How strong are those departments?

7. Are teaching fellows (usually graduate students or highly successful junior/senior students) involved in lecture(s) or lab work? Are they responsible for individual grading?

8. What are the "core course" and "liberal arts" course requirements at the school? How many credit hours and in what areas? (*e.g.* humanities, social sciences, computer science, psychology, philosophy, religion, etc.) Are there adequate course selections in those areas? How strong are those respective departments?

9. What are the class sizes like? Are the introductory premed courses taught in large lecture halls with hundreds of students? If they are, do these large courses break up into smaller "sections" to discuss lectures and problem sets? Are the introductory courses taught as smaller/lecture groups (usually 10-50 students)? Who are the faculty members that teach these courses? Who are the better instructors?

10. Is there a sufficient number of class positions available in courses that I will select for my major, premedical, or core course requirements?

11. If pre-registration is possible, how far in advance? If I don't pre-register for a certain course and decide to take it later, will I be able to get into that course?

12. Is there an Honors program or honor's track with regard to my major or other course selections?

13. If I major in a science, do I have a choice of obtaining either a B.A. or a B.S.? If there is a B.S. option, what are the additional requirements for the major?

14. Is there sufficient scheduling flexibility at the school? Is the same course taught at different times of the day or week (Monday, Wednesday, Friday vs. Tuesday/Thursday lectures)? Are evening classes available? How popular are they with undergraduate students?

15. Is there sufficient course availability/flexibility so that a class (*e.g.* Chemistry I or Biology I) is also offered in the second semester and not just the first semester?

16. What are the academic course policies on "withdrawals" and "incompletes"?

17. Is it possible to repeat a course if you, at first, receive a low grade?

18. Are the faculty readily accessible? What are their office hours and availability during the week (one day/week, two times/week, etc.)? Are teachers readily available right after lecture to ask a few questions or to do a problem(s)? Will a faculty member be willing to set up appointments with individual students or groups of students if they have additional questions or problems with a course?

19. Is tutoring (volunteer or paid) available in courses (especially science and math)?

20. What are summer sessions like if I choose to do coursework at that time? Length of a summer session(s)? What are the typical courses offered during these sessions?

21. Do tenured faculty teach at all levels of coursework. . . introductory, intermediate, advanced (graduate school)?

22. How are students typically graded?—exams, labs, problem sets, attendance, special projects, papers, etc.?

23. What types of exams are given? (Multiple choice, essay, short answer, problem-set type tests, etc.) Is there a scheduled weekly quiz? Are there surprise ("pop") quizzes?

2. SCHOOL'S REPUTATION AND PRESTIGE

1. National reputation and prestige?

2. Regional/local reputation?

3. Student body SAT scores/ACT scores: Average, median, range of scores (Median: 50% above this number and 50% below this number); SAT/ACT score range (usually given in the percentile range: 25%ile - 75%ile). Percentage of Freshman class who graduated in the top ten percent of their high school class.

4. Attrition rates/number of students dropping out or transferring?

5. Percentage of students who graduate in four years?

6. Percentage of students who take a leave of absence? Primary reasons for taking them?

7. What is the average number of students who declare themselves as "premed" during the freshman year? What is the attrition rate for these premeds by sophomore year/junior year/senior year?

8. Success of getting applicants into an allopathic (M.D.) medical school?

9. Any special arrangements with one or more medical schools? (*e.g.* early assurance or accelerated programs.)

10. Success rates of getting into an allopathic (M.D.) medical school with a non-science major? What are those successful majors? (*e.g.* history, economics, political science, philosophy, psychology, etc.)

11. Does the school have a post-baccalaureate program for college graduates who decide to apply to medical school?

12. Is the college's reputation based more on the quality of its graduate/professional schools?

13. What is the basis for the school's reputation? *e.g.* liberal arts; engineering; arts and humanities; allied health sciences (nursing, physical therapy, nutrition, pharmacy, etc.).

14. Is there a medical school affiliated with the college or university campus? How successful are the students in gaining admission to their university's medical school?

3. ACADEMIC AND PERSONAL COUNSELING/GRADUATE, PROFESSIONAL SCHOOL, AND JOB PLACEMENT

1. Are advisors assigned from freshman through senior year?

2. Premedical advisory system. How is it actually set up?

3. Adjunct services and resources for medical school applicants? (*e.g.* mock interviews, accessibility to MCAT preparation courses, etc.)

4. Is there more than one premed advisor? If needed, can I choose or change my advisor?

5. Adequate help in placing premed students in summer fellowships?

6. For unsuccessful medical school applicants or for those students taking time off before applying or going to medical school—is there good graduate school placement or job placement in an area applicable to health care or the basic medical sciences?

4. GEOGRAPHICAL AREA

1. Region of the country?

2. Particular city or state.

3. Hometown school or "somewhat local" (still able to commute from home).

4. City location vs. suburban vs. rural area.

5. "College town" atmosphere?

6. Close to cultural, sports, or recreational opportunities?

5. CAMPUS FACILITIES

1. Are there adequate lecture hall facilities?

2. Are the labs up-to-date?

3. Is there a "well-stocked" bookstore?

4. Library—what are its hours? Sufficient hours on weekends?

5. Are there "late at night" safe places to study on campus?

6. Campus parking: Cost? Accessibility to facilities?

7. Security: police/security officers; availability of student escort services to dorms and parking lots?

8. Does the school have more than one campus? Is there a shuttle bus service available?

6. EXTRACURRICULAR ACTIVITIES

1. Is there a premed club? Is it an active organization? What opportunities and activities does it provide?

2. Are there appropriate and beneficial premed activities available? (*e.g.* physician mentor programs or health-related volunteering.)

3. Activities that match your interests: *e.g.* sports, drama, debate, religious, music, social, etc.

4. Fraternities/sororities on campus?

7. COSTS/FINANCIAL AID

1. Tuition, room and board.

2. Other student fees.

3. Average semester book costs?

4. Accessibility to used books?

5. Are dorms available freshman through senior year?

6. Off-campus housing costs?

7. Scholarship and loan availability?

8. Student employment: adequate work-study arrangements?

8. OTHER IMPORTANT PERSONAL MATTERS

1. Availability of student health insurance plans.

2. Personal/psychological/psychiatric counseling services availability.

3. Good student health service? How close are hospitals, clinics, or doctors' offices?

4. Job availability for spouse.

5. Child care services?

6. Available campus housing for married students?

7. Availability of cafeteria menu plans for commuter or off-campus students.

And Finally . . .
Other Questions to Add to Your List

1. Will I be able to do any type of internship in my field or related area of interest? (summer vs. academic year, paid vs. volunteer, credit vs. non-credit)

2. What are the opportunities for undergraduates to serve as research assistants in a medically related area/specialty? Is this research done at a graduate school or a medical school?

3. If you desire on-campus housing for four years, can this be guaranteed?

4. By what semester and by what academic year are you required to declare your major? How easy is it to change majors?

5. Is there any type of crime on campus? How safe are the surrounding neighborhoods of

the campus? What is the crime rate for the city or community where the school is located?

Remember, no school will be absolutely perfect, but you can be well informed in choosing the school that's right for you. Deciding on which college to attend should never be a mystery. Well-informed college applicants can be pretty confident about choosing the right school once the "college acceptances start rolling in."

These aforementioned lists provide a myriad of factors and questions which should be considered when deciding what COLLEGE IS RIGHT FOR YOU! It is a detailed listing, but it really serves two purposes: First, these are factors that some students might not think about or even be aware of until they would actually attend that school. Secondly, these listed factors can provide good "food for thought"—they can serve to make you ask your own personal questions about the RIGHT SCHOOL FOR YOU!

Where can you get the answers to your questions? There are a variety of ways to find this information and the following "pearls of advice" should help you to guide your way through the maze of college applications, admissions, and your ultimate acceptance decision: (Note: The Resource Directory at the end of this chapter lists numerous outside sources which can help in the complex process of CHOOSING THE RIGHT SCHOOL FOR YOU.)

1. There are some very good reasonably priced college guides which provide good summary descriptions and addresses of colleges and universities across the country. What's more, schools are rated and ranked according to different factors (*e.g.* faculty, selectivity, financial resources, student retention rates, alumni contributions, etc.) along with a survey which is sent to several thousand college administrators. Remember, do not become obsessed with the numbers and the rankings. After you have assembled all the relative information about a school, you have to come up with YOUR OWN RANK LIST. . . . This is the list THAT REALLY COUNTS!

2. There are more voluminous college guides which give detailed information about each individual college or university. (Remember, that does not mean you have to load your bookshelves with these college guide compendiums. . . . Choosing one of these books will more than suffice; in fact, a good high school guidance office should have some of these various publications for you to begin your research.)

3. The good thing about most of these college admission guidebooks is that besides detailed descriptions of the individual schools, there are numerous articles on a vast array of topics covering both college admissions and that of selecting a college.

Examples of these topics may include:

1. Writing your application essay(s)

2. Early application process

3. Financial aid: scholarships/loans/student employment

4. ROTC: military scholarships

5. SAT preparation books

6. SAT preparatory courses

7. High school teacher recommendations

8. Social life on campus

9. Extracurricular activities

10. Participation in intercollegiate athletics

11. Career planning/job placement

12. Community colleges (two year junior colleges)

13. Filling out financial aid forms

14. Obtaining quality education at bargain tuition prices

4. Be aware of the various RANK LISTS used by these guidebooks. There are rankings which are subdivided into various categories. These schools may be listed under one or more categories: universities (national vs. regional), liberal arts colleges (national vs. regional), engineering, business, arts, "best dollar-value" schools, and schools with the largest and the least individual student-debt loads.

5. College guides will also give you detailed information and statistics on a variety of categories which may include some of the following: application deadlines/expenses/ financial aid/freshman admission information/type of academic calendar/information on class size, undergraduate student body, and "most popular majors" at that school.

6. An excellent way of finding out specific information that you would like answered is to write to the Freshman Dean's Office, the Admissions Office, or the Dean of Students. These offices are very good at answering prospective students questions; furthermore, they can furnish you with names and addresses of important offices you should contact: *e.g.* the premed advisory office, career counseling, departments in which you might major, financial aid, etc. These are some of the offices that should be able to answer all of your specific questions regarding both your future undergraduate premedical and academic career.

7. Campus visits can be informative, especially if you do your homework ahead of time. Write ahead to schedule appointments with various offices (*e.g.* premed advising, academic departments in which you may later declare your major). This will usually mean that you will have to visit the campus on a weekday. . . . but it will be worth it—remember, this is an investment in both your academic and professional future. By visiting the prospective schools—the ones you are really interested in attending and have a good chance of admission—you will be given the opportunity to do a variety of activities: campus and library tours, visiting labs and lecture halls, talking to students, visiting classes, staying in a dorm overnight, etc. Staying on campus for more than a day will also give you excellent contacts—your host student(s) will be able to introduce you to premed students and also those students in your prospective major(s). Spend some time with these students. . . . Talk to them! . . . They are the ones who can give you a true perspective "on being premed" at that particular school.

8. Use a variety of prospective personal resources that you might not have previously considered: Alumni from your high school may be attending or have graduated from that college you are considering. How about students from other high schools who were involved in some of the same extracurricular activities (*e.g.* sports, debate, etc.) and are now attending a college/university that interests you? What about family friends or neighborhood friends? . . . Some may have a son or daughter attending a school that you are seriously considering. Do not hesitate to use these potential contacts. . . . If you are going to make a four-year investment in time, energy, and tuition, you do want to make the right decision.

To conclude this chapter, I have provided a list of outside resources that cover a number of areas regarding your future college years. This list is detailed, but it provides a variety of books that cover these areas in a comprehensive manner. If you do your research carefully, you will be able to find them in libraries, large bookstores, and guidance/college counseling offices. Parents will also find these resources enlightening as they help their children through their college years.

These outside resources have been divided into the following areas: (There are also some introductory resources providing an overview of college admissions and college life.)

1. College Admissions

2. College Directories

3. College Experience (General)

4. College Application Essays

5. Financial Aid

6. Campus Visits/Interviews

7. College Majors

8. Study Skills/Test-Taking

9. Parents' References

10. Internship Programs

11. Adult Students Returning to College

Introductory Resources

Time/The Princeton Review's *The Best College for You and How to Get In,* (updated annually).

U.S. News and World Report, *America's Best Colleges.* Washington, DC, (updated annually).

Outside Resources

1. COLLEGE ADMISSIONS

1. Adler. *100 Colleges Where Average Students Can Excel.* New York, NY: Macmillan Reference, a Simon and Schuster Macmillan Company, 1996.

2. Antonoff, Steven R. *The College Finder.* New York: Ballantine Books, 1993.

3. Frank, Steven, Fred Zuker, Alice Murphey, and the Staff of the Kaplan Educational Centers. *The Road to College: Expert Advice for Navigating the Admissions Process,* 1998 Edition. New York, NY: Kaplan Educational Centers and Simon and Schuster, 1997.

4. _____, and Marie Friedemann. *College Match: A Blueprint for Choosing the Best School for You!* 4th edition. Alexandria, VA: Octameron Associates, 1995.

5. Kaplan Educational Centers, Staff of. *Get Into College Toolkit.* New York, NY: Simon and Schuster, 1997.

6. Ordovensky, Pat. *USA Today: Peterson's Getting into College.* Princeton, NJ: Peterson's and Gannett New Media Services, 1995.

7. Pope, Loren. *Looking Beyond the Ivy League: Finding the College That's Right for You.* New York, NY: Penguin Books, 1995.

8. _____. *Colleges That Change Lives: 40 Schools You Should Know About Even if You're Not a Straight-A Student.* New York, NY: Penguin Books, 1996.

9. Robinson, Adam and John Katzman, eds. *The Princeton Review Student Advantage Guide to College Admissions.* New York, NY: Random House, Inc., 1996.

10. Unger, Harlow. *A Student's Guide to College Admissions: Everything Your Guidance Counselor Has No Time to Tell You.* 3rd edition. New York, NY: Facts on File, Inc., 1995.

11. Wolff, Michael ed. *How to Get Into the School of Your Dreams Using the Internet and Online Services.* New York, NY: New Media L.L.C., 1996.

2. COLLEGE DIRECTORIES

1. Ahmad, S. *The Yale Daily News Guide to Succeeding in College.* New York, NY: Kaplan Educational Centers and Simon and Schuster, 1997.

2. ARCO. *The Right College.* 7th edition. New York, NY: ARCO Publishing, a Division of Simon and Schuster, Inc., 1994.

3. Cass - Liepmann, Julia ed. *Cass and Birnbaum's Guide to American Colleges.* 17th edition. Scranton, PA: HarperCollins, Inc., 1996.

4. College Division of Barron's Educational Series ed. *Barron's Compact Guide to Colleges.* 10th edition. Hauppauge, NY: Barron's Educational Series, Inc., 1996.

5. _____. *Barron's Profiles of American Colleges, Descriptions of the Colleges.* 22nd Edition. Hauppauge, NY: Barron's Educational Series, Inc., 1997.

6. *The College Handbook, 1998.* New York, NY: College Board Publications, 1997.

7. Custard, Edward, and Dan Saraceno. *The Princeton Review: The Complete Book of Catholic Colleges, 1998 Edition.* New York, NY: Random House, Inc. and Princeton Review Publishing L.L.C., 1997.

8. _____, John Katzman, Tom Meltzer, and Zachary Knowler. *The Princeton Review Student Advantage Guide to the Best 311 Colleges.* New York, NY: Random House, Inc. and Princeton Review Publishing L.L.C., 1997.

9. Fischgrund, Tom ed. *Barron's Top 50: An Inside Look at America's Best Colleges.* 3rd edition. Hauppauge, NY: Barron's Educational Series Inc., 1995.

10. Fiske, Edward B. *The Fiske Guide to Colleges.* 14th edition. New York, NY: Time Books, a Division of Random House, Inc., 1997.

11. Kaplan Educational Centers. *The College Catalog.* New York, NY: Kaplan Educational Centers and Simon and Schuster, 1996.

12. *Peterson's Competitive Colleges, 1997-1998.* 16th edition. Princeton, NJ: Peterson's, 1997.

13. *Peterson's Competitive Colleges, 1996-1997: Top Colleges for Top Students.* 15th edition. Princeton, NJ: Peterson's, 1996.

14. *Peterson's Guide to Four-Year Colleges.* 28th edition. Princeton, NJ: Peterson's, 1997.

15. Straughn, Barbara Lovejoy, and Charles T. Straughn II. *Lovejoy's College Guide.* 23rd edition. New York, NY: Macmillan, a Simon and Schuster Macmillan Company, 1995.

16. Yale Daily News, The Staff of. *The Insider's Guide to the Colleges.* Griffin, NY: St. Martin's, 1997.

(Be aware that many of these college directories are updated annually or every two/three years.)

3. COLLEGE EXPERIENCE (GENERAL)

1. Carter, Carol. *Majoring in the Rest of Your Life: Career Secrets for College Students.* New York, NY: The Noonday Press, 1995.

2. DiYanni, Robert. *The Insider's Guide to College Success.* Needham Heights, MA: Allyn and Bacon, 1997.

3. Gottesman, Greg, and Friends. *College Survival.* 4th edition. New York, NY: ARCO, Macmillan General Reference, 1996.

4. Grayson, Paul and Philip Meilman. *Beating the College Blues.* New York, NY: Facts on File, Inc., 1992.

5. Hall, Colin, and Don Lieber. *Taking Time Off: Inspiring Stories of Students Who Enjoyed Successful Breaks from College and How You Can Plan Your Own.* New York, NY: The Noonday Press, 1996.

6. Ragins, M. *Making the Most of Your College Education.* New York, NY: An Owl Book, Henry Holt and Co., 1996.

7. Sponholz, Melanie, and Joseph Sponholz. *The Princeton Review College Companion: Real Students, True Stories, Good Advice.* New York, NY: Random House, Inc. and Princeton Review Publishing L.L.C., 1996.

8. Worthington, Janet, and Ronald Farrar. *The Ultimate College Survival Guide.* Princeton, NJ: Peterson's, 1995.

4. COLLEGE APPLICATION ESSAYS

1. Bauld, Harry. *On Writing the College Application Essay.* Harper and Row Publishers, 1987.

2. Curry, Boykin, and Brian Kasbar. *Essays that Worked: 50 Essays from Successful Applications to the Nation's Top Colleges.* New York: Fawcett Columbine, 1990.

3. Davidson, Wilma, and Susan McCloskey. *Writing a Winning College Application Essay.* Princeton, NJ: Peterson's, 1996.

4. Georges, Christopher J., and Gigi Georges and Staff Members of the Harvard Independent. *100 Successful College Application Essays.* New York, NY: A Mentor Book, Penguin Books, 1988.

5. Mason, Michael. *How to Write a Winning College Application Essay.* 2nd edition. Rocklin, CA: Prima Publishing, 1994.

6. Nourse, Kenneth A. *How to Write Your College Application Essay.* Lincolnwood, Illinois: VGM Career Horizons, 1996.

7. Power and DiAntonio. *The Admissions Essay: How to Stop Worrying and Start Writing!* New York, NY: Carol Publishing Group, 1995.

8. Van Raalte, Susan D. *College Applications and Essays.* 3rd edition. New York, NY: Arco, Macmillan General Reference, 1993.

5. FINANCIAL AID

1. ARCO. *College Scholarships and Financial Aid (With Arco's Scholarship Search Software).* 6th edition. New York, NY: An Arco Book, Macmillan General Reference, 1995.

2. Bellantoni, Patrick L. *College Financial Aid Made Easy.* Berkeley, CA: Ten Speed Press, 1996.

3. Blum, Laurie. *Free Money for College.* 4th edition. New York, NY: Facts on File, Inc., 1996.

4. Cassidy, Daniel. *The Scholarship Book.* Englewood Cliffs, NJ: Prentice-Hall, Inc., 1990.

5. The College Board. *College Costs and Financial Aid Handbook.* New York, NY: The College Board, 1997.

6. Davis, Kristin. *Financing College.* Washington, DC: Kiplinger Books, 1996.

7. Dennis, Marguerite J. *Barron's Complete College Financing Guide.* 4th edition. Hauppauge, NY: Barron's Educational Series, Inc., 1997.

8. Deutschman, Alan. *Winning Money for College.* 3rd edition. Princeton, NJ: Peterson's Guides, 1992.

9. Hastings, Penny, and Todd Caven. *How to Win a Sports Scholarship.* Los Angeles, CA: First Base Sports, Inc., 1995.

10. Jaffe, David. *The New College Financial Aid System: Making It Work for You.* Tulsa, OK: Council Oak Books, 1993.

11 Kaplan Educational Centers. *Scholarships: The Essential Guide, 1997-1998 Edition.* New York, NY: Kaplan Educational Centers and Simon and Schuster, 1996.

12. Leider, Anna, and Robert Leider. *Don't Miss Out: The Ambitious Student's Guide to Financial Aid.* 21st edition. Alexandria, VA: Octameron Associates, Inc., 1996.

13. *Less Competitive College Grants and Loans.* 2nd edition. Houston, TX: Student College Aid, 1995.

14. McKee, Cynthia R., and Phillip McKee Jr. *Cash for College.* New York, NY: Hearst Books, William Morrow and Company, Inc., 1993.

15. Murphey, Alice, and the Staff of the Kaplan Educational Centers. *You Can Afford College: The Family Guide to Meeting College Costs.* New York, NY: Kaplan Educational Centers and Simon and Schuster, 1996.

16. Ordovensky, Pat. *Financial Aid for College.* Princeton, NJ: Peterson's, 1995.

17. Ragins, Marianne. *Winning Scholarships for College: An Insider's Guide.* New York, NY: Henry Holt and Co., Inc., 1994.

18. Rosenwasser, Edward. *How to Obtain Maximum College Financial Aid.* 4th edition. Houston, TX: Student College Aid Publishing Division, 1994.

19. Smith. *Money Magazine: Paying for Your Child's College Education.* New York, NY: Warner Books, Inc., 1996.

20. Student Services, Inc. *The Complete Scholarship Book.* Naperville, Illinois: Sourcebooks, Inc., 1996.

21. Walker, Ron ed. *Peterson's Sports Scholarships and College Athletic Programs.* Princeton, NJ: Peterson's Guides, Inc., 1996.

6. CAMPUS VISITS/ INTERVIEWS

1. Fry, Ronald. *Your First Interview.* 3rd edition. Franklin Lakes, NJ: Career Press, 1996.

2. _____. *Your First Resume.* 4th edition. Franklin Lakes, NJ: Career Press, 1996.

3. Schneider, Zola D. *Campus Visits and College Interviews.* New York, NY: The College Board, 1987.

4. Spencer, Jane, and Sandra Maleson. *The Princeton Review Student Advantage Guide to Visiting College Campuses.* New York, NY: Random House, Inc., 1996.

7. COLLEGE MAJORS

1. *The College Board Guide to 150 Popular Majors.* New York, NY: College Board Publications (Published/revised annually).

2. Digby, Joan. *Peterson's Honors Programs.* Princeton, NJ: Peterson's, 1997.

3. Garcia, John. *Majoring in Engineering: How to Get from Your Freshman Year to Your First Job.* New York, NY: The Noonday Press, 1995.

4. *Index of Majors and Graduate Degrees.* New York, NY: College Board Publications. (Published/revised annually)

8. STUDY SKILLS/TEST-TAKING

1. Armstrong, William. *Study Tactics.* Hauppauge, NY: Barron's Educational Series, Inc., 1983.

2. Johnson, Susan. *Taking the Anxiety Out of Taking Tests.* Oakland, CA: New Harbinger Publications, Inc., 1997.

3. Robinson, Adam. *What Smart Students Know: Maximum Grades, Optimum Learning, Minimum Time.* New York, NY: Crown Publishers, Inc., 1993.

9. PARENTS' REFERENCES

1. Borden, M.E. and M.A. Burlinson and E.R. Kearns. *In Addition to Tuition: The Parents Survival Guide to Freshman Year of College.*
New York, NY: Facts on File, Inc., 1995.

2. Boyer, Ernest L., and Paul Boyer. *Smart Parents Guide to Colleges: The 10 Most Important Factors When Choosing a College.* Princeton, NJ: Peterson's, 1996.

3. Coburn, Karen L., and M.L. Treeger. *Letting Go: A Parent's Guide to Today's College Experience.* Bethesda, MD: Adler and Adler Publishers, Inc., 1992.

4. Hayden, Thomas C. *Peterson's Handbook for College Admissions: The Essential Family Guide to Selecting Colleges, Visits and Interviews, Applications, Financial Aid: The Freshman Year.* 4th Edition. Princeton, NJ: Peterson's, 1995.

5. MacGowan, Sandra, and Sarah McGinty. *50 College Admission Directors Speak to Parents.* New York, NY: Harcourt, Brace, Jovanovich, 1988.

6. Rubenstone, Sally, and Sidonia Dalby. *College Admissions: A Crash Course for Panicked Parents.* New York, NY: Arco, Macmillan General Reference, 1994.

7. Shields, Charles J. *The College Guide for Parents.* 3rd edition. New York, NY: The College Entrance Examination Board, 1995.

10. INTERNSHIP PROGRAMS

1. Bauer, Betsy. *Getting Work Experience: The Student's Directory of Professional Internship Programs.* New York, NY: Dell Publishing Group.

2. Gilbert, Sara D. *ARCO Internships: A Directory for Career-Finders.* New York, NY: Macmillan, Inc., 1995.

3. Oldman, Mark, and Samer Hamadeh. *The Princeton Review, America's Top Internships, 1998 Edition.* New York, NY: Random House, Inc. and Princeton Review Publishing L.L.C., 1997.

11. ADULT STUDENTS
RETURNING TO COLLEGE

1. Bruno, Frank J. *Going Back to School: College Survival Strategies for Adult Students.* New York, NY: ARCO, Macmillan General Reference, 1995.

2. Ludden, Laverne L., and Marsha J. Ludden. *Luddens' Adult Guide to Colleges and Universities.* Indianapolis, IN: Park Avenue Productions, 1997.

6

"Signs and Symptoms of Being Premed": Accentuating the Positive and Avoiding the Negative

Countless words and descriptions have been used over the years to describe premedical students. The "negative descriptions", unfortunately, are many: "too overly competitive," "hyper," "cutthroat," "wonks," "too narrow- minded and focused," "grade-greedy" (a/k/a "grade grubbing"), an "A" at "any cost," an "A" or "nothing," "absolute and total OVERACHIEVERS", "obsessive-compulsive" or a "totally me person." At the same time, however, the positive characteristics of premedical students have also been well described: highly motivated and disciplined, "well-organized," idealistic, intelligent, brilliant, and empathetic.

What occurs too often is that to "the outside world" (non-medical people), the negative characteristics overwhelm the "positive attributes." One of the most bothersome terms used has been that of the "incessant overachiever." To counteract that particular negative connotation, one simply has to ask the opposite "question": WHO WANTS TO BE AN UNDERACHIEVER? . . . "I certainly do not!" The harsh reality is that no matter what the job or profession, an "underachiever" falls short of his/her goal.

No matter what your "intellect" may be or academic background, it does take over-achievement to get through medical school. Those who disparagingly use the "o" word ("overachiever") have neither been to medical school nor know what it really takes to get through the rigors of medical school. Most high school students are probably fully aware of who the underachiever(s) really are. These are the students who "ace" the SAT exam (scores of 1200 or higher) but who get mediocre grades. These students may outscore the "top ten" of the class in terms of their SAT scores, but in terms of college admissions, top schools are not "knocking down their doors" because of their otherwise average or "subpar" performance. At the same time, these "underachievers" can become very frustrated when they see the valedictorian or salutatorian obtain admission into an Ivy League school with a SAT score "lower than their score." The natural reaction by underachievers is obvious: "If only I had studied harder; if only I had taken my high school years more seriously! . . . These students are, "after the fact," disappointed with their high school performances.

The good news is that whether you are an "overachiever" or an "underachiever," it is never too late to set your sights on medical school. Remember, not every high school valedictorian or salutatorian or "top ten" student gets into medical school. Any student who "simply rests on his/her high school laurels or relies on a top premedical university's reputation alone will not gain admission into medical school. If you were an underachiever in high school, you can turn it all the way around in college. . . . You know you have the intellectual talent. . . . Now, just APPLY YOURSELF! Unless you are in a six or seven-year medical school program (where high school grades are a factor), your high school record will not matter. . . . It is what you DO NOW. . . . It all comes down to how you are NOW performing in college (and you don't even have to be at that "top 50" college or university). Some students complain that they were "not challenged" in high school or were "not particularly motivated" to do well. These students usually state that they were not willing to put forth the effort because they really didn't know their interests nor ever found "their real niche." Again, the good news is THAT WAS HIGH SCHOOL. . . . Medical schools look at how you ARE PERFORMING NOW! If you are now motivated to become a doctor and are willing to put forth the appropriate effort. . . Whatever you did/however you PERFORMED in HIGH SCHOOL is well. . . HISTORY! On the other hand, if you are a student who did well in high school and was disciplined and highly motivated. . . "continue those ATTRIBUTES," and you should continue to be highly successful.

The harsh reality of premedicine is that the number of medical school applications is by far exceeding the number of available first-year positions. This trend will not change in the near future. . . .   On the average, there are two to three unsuccessful applicants for every one student who will be admitted to the following first-year class. The fact that qualified medical school applicants are rejected every year only seems to "ever intensify" premedical competition at the collegiate level. What's more, the demographics of every matriculating medical school class has been constantly changing since the 1980s: No longer is the "standard admittee" white, male, and 22 years of age. With a seemingly ever increase in both the absolute number and variety of backgrounds (ethnic/racial/gender/socioeconomic) in the applicant pool, the competition is both STIFF and INTENSE; even students with "A-" to "A" averages and very good MCAT scores sometimes do not get admitted to medical school.

Unfortunately, those who "suffer from the negative signs and symptoms of being premed (those characteristics mentioned earlier in the chapter) fall earlier into a trap which I call the "hypocrisy of premedicine." This trap becomes hypocrisy because ALL THOSE GREAT IDEALS it takes to be admitted to medical school (and eventually become a compassionate physician) seemingly FALL BY THE WAYSIDE. These characteristics that relate to "success at any cost" need to be "toned down to a minimal" or "totally removed." Having a "kinder and gentler premed student body" may seem to be too idealistic, but it is a MOVE IN THE RIGHT DIRECTION! . . . Creating excessive amounts of self-created stress/anxiety/tension can only work to debilitate otherwise healthy physical, emotional, and mental states.

As a premedical student, you should REALIZE EARLY that it does take "overachievement" to get through medical school—all of your faculties (physical/mental/emotional) will be tested to the "outer limits"; there is usually no way of appreciating this fact until you are actually in medical school. If you concentrate on accentuating the positive qualities of hard work, discipline, and delayed gratification, you will see that these same characteristics will help you during your entire life . . . from undergraduate school to medical school to residency . . . to a FULFILLING PROFESSIONAL CAREER.

There are also other qualities and characteristics that you should be "aware of" as you go from high school/college student to young medical professional. PERSONAL/PROFESSIONAL GROWTH AND DEVELOPMENT is a "continuous process"—no one can claim to have a monopoly on all of these ideal attributes . . . . Remember you cannot be "all things to all people" (and, of course, no one is perfect!). Many of these descriptions may seem obvious to the reader; they are listed here only to remind the reader that TRUE GROWTH cannot occur without the discovery of those ideals that he/she has the potential "to aspire to presently and for the future".

Accentuate the Positive Qualities/Characteristics/Descriptions... Those That Will Make You a Better Person and Physician

Integrity	Be Organized
Compassionate	Manage Your Time Well
Empathetic	Intelligent
Dedicated	Sense of Humor
Understanding	Hard Worker
Respectful	Positive Thinker/Optimistic
Caring	Ambitious
Delayed Gratification	Confident
Friendly	Exhibit Character
Humility	Perseverence
Capable of Good Judgement	Sincere

Enthusiastic

Patient

Self-Motivated

Dedicated to Serving Others

Flexibility

Conscientious

Genuinely Interested In People

Interested in Medicine as
Both a Science and an Art

Understand What It Means
to Be a Team Player.

Be a Leader

Mature

Good Imagination/Being Creative

Honesty

Truthful

Polite

Disciplined

Do Not Be an Underachiever
When You Can Be Capable
of so Much More

(Note: The above list is not in any particular order nor does it list every possible attribute.)

7

Premedical Course Scheduling

A wide variety of factors will determine how you schedule your premedical coursework in college. When you plan your course schedule every semester, keep the following general principles in mind:

1. There are numerous scheduling options which are available. These schedules are usually strongly suggested/recommended by the Premedical Advisory and/or Science (*e.g.* Biology) Departments at that particular school. At some schools, students are encouraged to take full year courses in mathematics, biology, and chemistry during their freshman year; other schools have their freshmen concentrate on finishing the mathematics and general chemistry requirements.

2. The student also has to look at his/her background in science and mathematics. If the student has a weak or average high school background, taking math, chemistry, and biology all in the freshman year would not be a good idea. (Remember TO STAY WITHIN YOURSELF. . . ONE SCHEDULE DOES NOT FIT ALL STUDENTS!) You do not want to be finished with your premedical studies even before you really get started! . . . Early science and math course "overloads" can prove to be "grade costly"!

3. When planning your schedules, always keep in mind the minimum credit hours needed to be considered a full-time student at your school. Also note the total number of credit hours required both in your major and to fulfill graduation requirements. For example, if you take the minimum number of credit hours for full-time status during the semester of your MCATs, you will have to offset that with a heavier schedule during another semester.

4. Know the available credit hours for fulfilling liberal arts college requirements. You may need to fulfill certain numbers of credit hours in such areas as humanities, social sciences, behavioral sciences, fine arts, philosophy, theology, etc.

5. Be aware of available credit hours for electives. It is important for you to choose both science and non-science course electives which interest you.

6. Another factor that will determine your science course load will be your major; obviously, non-science majors do not have to take as heavy of a science/math course load as their science major premedical counterparts. At the same time, however, non-science majors will have fewer chances to bolster their science GPA if they receive one or more poor grades.

7. Engineering and math majors will have more rigorous course loads. They will need to fulfill their science/math foundation courses early so that they can start taking more advanced courses for their major by their sophomore or junior year. As you can see, if you add in one biology course for the premedical requirement and at least one or more classes (*e.g.* physiology) for a good biology knowledge base, these majors will be "extremely busy."

8. The necessary credit hours in math (*e.g.* Calculus I and/or II) will also depend on your major's math requirements. Also note that while calculus is recommended by most medical schools, it is only required by approximately twenty percent of the schools.

9. Summer courses will also affect your semester course load and your course sequencing during the academic year. It is difficult to plan summer course schedules early in your college career. The need or opportunity to take summer courses is usually a personal choice and becomes easier to plan once you are in college for at least one year. Financial and time constraints may also limit this option.

10. Accelerated B.S. or B.A./M.D. programs (*e.g.* 6-7 years) have rigorous science course loads. (Up to three science/math courses every semester and mandatory summer courses.) Depending on the program, the student may be required to take more difficult basic science prerequisites (*e.g.* calculus-based physics courses).

11. The Bachelor of Science Degree option (Discussed in Chapter 8, "Selecting a Major") may require you to take up to three science/math courses every semester.

12. Depending on the department or the school, you may also be required to do a research project and/or a senior thesis.

To conclude this chapter, two sample schedules are provided as a guide for scheduling premedical coursework.

Sample I

FRESHMAN YEAR

First Semester	Credit Hours	Second Semester	Credit Hours
General Chemistry I (with lab)	4	General Chemistry II (with lab)	4
Mathematics: (1) Algebra/Trigonometry (2) Pre-Calculus or (3) Calculus I	3 - 4	Mathematics: (1) Algebra/Trigonometry (2) Pre-Calculus or (3) Calculus I or II	3 - 4
Liberal Arts/college requirements	4 - 5	Liberal Arts/college requirements	5 - 8
English (Composition or Literature)	3		
	14 - 16		12 - 16

Note:

1. If the student has a weak background in high school math and/or chemistry, it may be necessary to take Biology I instead of Chemistry I during the freshman year. Another possibility would be to not take biology and do remedial work (*e.g.* chemistry for non-premedical students may be a possibility in this situation).

2. If a student is considering a non-science major he/she can take some courses (*e.g.* humanities, social sciences, psychology) that may also fulfill a college/liberal arts requirement.

SOPHOMORE YEAR

First Semester	Credit Hours	Second Semester	Credit Hours
Biology I (with lab)	4	Biology II (with lab)	4
Organic Chemistry I (with lab)	4	Organic Chemistry II (with lab)	4
Liberal Arts/college requirements	2 - 5	Liberal Arts/college requirements	2 - 5
Major	4	Major	4
	14 - 17		14 - 17

If a student is still undecided about his/her major, there is still enough flexibility during the sophomore year to take courses which fulfill both a college requirement and a potential requirement for a major. (*e.g.* A student could take a history class and also fulfill a social science college requirement.)

JUNIOR YEAR

First Semester	Credit Hours	Second Semester	Credit Hours
Physics I (with lab)	4	Physics II (with lab)	4
Major/electives	12 - 14	Major/electives	12 - 14
	16 - 18		16 - 18

SENIOR YEAR

First Semester	Credit Hours	Second Semester	Credit Hours
Major/electives	14 - 17	Major/electives	14 - 17

Sample II

FRESHMAN YEAR

First Semester	Credit Hours	Second Semester	Credit Hours
Biology I (with lab)	4	Biology II (with lab)	4
General Chemistry I (with lab)	4	General Chemistry II (with lab)	4
Mathematics:	3 - 4	Mathematics:	3 - 4
(1) Algebra/Trigonometry or		(1) Algebra/Trigonometry	
(2) Pre-Calculus or		(2) Pre-Calculus or	
(3) Calculus I		(3) Calculus I or II	
English (Composition or Literature)	3	Liberal Arts/college requirements	4 - 5
	14 - 15		15 - 17

SOPHOMORE YEAR

First Semester	Credit Hours	Second Semester	Credit Hours
Organic Chemistry I (with lab)	4	Organic Chemistry II (with lab)	4
Liberal Arts/college requirements	6 - 9	Liberal Arts/college requirements	6 - 9
Major	4	Major	4
	14 - 17		14 - 17

JUNIOR YEAR

First Semester	Credit Hours	Second Semester	Credit Hours
Physics I (with lab)	4	Physics II (with lab)	4
Major/electives	12 - 14	Major/electives	12 - 14
	16 - 18		16 - 18

SENIOR YEAR

First Semester	Credit Hours	Second Semester	Credit Hours
Major/electives	14 - 18	Major electives	14 - 18

These are only two examples but they do serve as basic guidelines. There are, of course, a number of factors (discussed in detail in the first part of this chapter) that can affect the scheduling of certain courses. Depending on your academic background, you many need to take a course out of sequence (*e.g.* Chemistry I during the second semester [if offered]). Also, some schools may suggest physics during the sophomore year and organic chemistry during the junior year.

In conclusion, you should always do a personal reassessment every semester when planning your schedule. Besides the requirements for your major, you need to know your strengths, weaknesses, and educational goals in formulating an appropriate academic schedule.

8
Selecting A Major

The first major principle that premed students should follow is to major in an area that interests them. If you have a passion for science, then by all means, major in one of the biological or physical sciences. Some students even choose to major in an engineering science or mathematics. Avoid the mistake of majoring in an area of science ONLY TO APPLY to medical school.

What's more, who wants to be "miserable" majoring in an area that does not really interest them. Remember, you are investing TIME, TUITION, and ENERGY. . . . Invest WISELY by choosing the RIGHT MAJOR FOR YOU! No matter what your major may be, make sure that you challenge yourself intellectually and develop a work ethic that will pay off once you are in medical school.

Majoring in a Biological Science Discipline

BIOLOGY (biology, zoology, microbiology, genetics, biochemistry)

Majoring in biology at your particular college or university may add difficulty to your program because premeds tend to congregate to this major. If you see yourself both as a biology major (because you are genuinely interested in the subject matter) and an "able bodied student" ready to face intense competition over the next four years, then you have found the right major (GO FOR IT!). If you do major in biology, you will be able to gain an added advantage for medical school if you take the appropriate undergraduate courses. If your department does not require you to take any course(s) in the areas of botany, marine biology, ecology, or environmental science, do not take them. If you, however, do have a genuine interest in one of these areas, then by all means, take the course(s); you could also use such coursework as a foundation for an alternative career (botanist, marine biologist, etc.) if you decide not to attend medical school. If they do require you to take some of these courses, you may want to take the minimal number. . . . Why?. . . . Coursework in human biology and animal science will give you an ADVANTAGE in medical school. (This advantage will become apparent especially in your first year when you will be so overwhelmed with your new voluminous

---

workload; the second year of medical school contains even more material, but by that time you should be acclimated to the expectations of medical school.)

What are these "advantageous courses"? Physiology and biochemistry are two major courses during the first year in medical school that will take up much of your class and study time. At most medical schools, these courses are considered full-year courses and will be taught each semester (or each trimester, depending on the academic schedule). Other medical school courses such as histology, genetics, and embryology "do pack in voluminous amounts of material" but are not taught over the course of a full year. Most undergraduate colleges will have course offerings in histology/embryology and genetics, so see if you can fit some of them into your schedule. One or more of these courses could be taken during your senior year when the material will be "fresh" for the start of medical school.

Taking two or more of these courses (especially physiology and biochemistry) as an undergraduate will help make your workload more manageable in medical school. The content may not be as voluminous or as detailed as in medical school, but it will give you more than an adequate introduction to the course expectations as a future medical student. (You will not, however, be able to substitute these undergraduate courses for the ones in medical school.) Doing well in these course(s) will also show evidence of your science aptitude.

Other courses that would give you a distinct advantage are either vertebrate anatomy or gross (human) anatomy. Vertebrate anatomy ("comparative vertebrate anatomy" or sometimes known as "verts") has the reputation of being one of the toughest courses in any undergraduate school to get an "A." I have met students in medical school who received a "C" in "verts" as undergraduates; most of these students felt, however, that the time and academic investment in this course paid off when taking gross anatomy in medical school. They all seemed to have an excellent grasp of the musculoskeletal system, one of the areas that is usually covered very early in medical school anatomy. The "average" gross anatomy (human) course is offered by relatively few undergraduate schools but will only cover a small percentage of what you will be expected to know in medical school. More "intense" gross anatomy courses are sometimes taught as a cooperative effort between a medical school and an undergraduate department (*e.g.* Physical Therapy [PT] or Occupational Therapy [OT]). These courses are sometimes taught in the summer and are taken as prerequisites for continuing in that particular discipline (OT or PT). They will have much more detail than any "average" undergraduate gross anatomy class and will be the "closest thing" to an actual first-year med school course. They also tend to be extremely competitive (sometimes even more than organic chemistry) because, unfortunately, they act to "weed out" students who hope to become physical or occupational therapists.

Allied Health Professionals

There are some students who plan on careers in other health-related areas (*e.g.* nursing, nutrition, pharmacy, physical therapy) and then decide to go to medical school later in their college years or after they have been working in their chosen field. Any person falling into this category must carefully check their undergraduate science classes to see if individual courses fulfill premedical requirements. Many times, allied health students or professionals must take further work in the basic sciences (chemistry, physics, and biology) because course requirements for their major did not include "premed caliber" type classes. For example, many of these students may have taken "Introduction to Chemistry" or basic physics but the course content was not as difficult as those courses taken to fulfill the premed requirements. Each of the basic science departments usually offers a less rigorous introductory course; make sure that if you switch to a premed curriculum, that you take the appropriate introductory basic science coursework. Course catalogs or departmental brochures usually have detailed descriptions of their individual courses. With introductory courses, it is very common to see one of the following descriptions: "This course fulfills a basic science medical school admissions requirement." Alternatively, you may see this description: "This course does not fulfill an admissions requirement for medical school." If the course has the latter description, an added note will usually depict the course name and number which does fulfill the requirement. If these descriptions are not evident from either course catalogs or brochures, the student should go directly to a premed advisor or to the departmental office to find information on the appropriate courses.

Majoring in the Physical Sciences (Chemistry or Physics)/ Engineering/or Mathematics

These are the "thinking man's/woman's" majors. Rote memorization and regurgitation of facts and figures will simply not get you through any of these disciplines. Students who DO VERY WELL ACADEMICALLY IN ONE OF THESE MAJORS are respected by fellow students, faculty members, and yes, medical school admissions committees. Succeeding in one of these disciplines proves that the student is a "problem solver," a "critical thinker," and has an "analytical mind"—all descriptions that bode well with these same committee members. Doing very well in these majors also demonstrates an ability to handle difficult science/mathematical coursework and shows that you have the potential to succeed in the "basic science" medical school curriculum. If you are an "intuitive thinker" and can "think like a chemist, physicist, engineer, or mathematician," one of these majors may be for you. As an alternative, if your medical school plans change, these majors usually translate into very marketable skills (especially engineering and math; it may be necessary to seek a M.S. or Ph.D. degree in chemistry or physics to be really marketable). In choosing such a major, the overriding principle still stands: YOU MUST GENUINELY LIKE YOUR MAJOR! This will be "your academic life" for your undergraduate years, so you should enjoy what you do. This principle is especially important for anyone who decides to major in one of the aforementioned disciplines. When you choose one of these majors, keep in mind that your hopes for a broad based premedical or liberal education will be much more limited than the average student. You will also be carrying a heavier and more difficult science course load than even the average biology major. Taking two to three science/engineering/mathematics courses to fulfill both your major's requirements and the premedical curriculum will become your normal schedule. These majors all require other foundation courses such as advanced math (calculus III/"differential equations and beyond"), computer science, and statistics. Add up all of your other advanced course requirements for your major (*e.g.* A chemistry major usually requires, at a minimum, advanced organic chemistry, quantitative analysis, and physical chemistry), and as you can see, you will be extremely busy.

Succeeding at such an ambitious goal is possible, but you must be keenly aware of both the potential benefits and drawbacks. By majoring in one of these disciplines, most of your medical school admissions requirements (except biology) will be fulfilled automatically because many of these majors require introductory chemistry, physics, and mathematics courses.

One of the biggest challenges in majoring in one of these areas and being premed is the potential lost opportunity for taking one or more additional upper division biology courses (*e.g.* physiology, biochemistry, histology/embryology). These are the courses that will have a definite, positive influence on your time-management skills during your first year of medical school. If you are a chemistry, physics, engineering, or math major, these upper level biological courses will also help develop your rote memorization skills. Many non-biological science majors who enter medical school tell of being in "study shock"—overwhelmed by the seemingly incomprehensible volume of material to be covered; memorization skills (which can be further developed by taking upper level biology courses appropriate for medical school—*e.g.* physiology, biochemistry, histology/embryology, microbiology, human anatomy, vertebrate anatomy) can serve as a major lifeline for surviving medical school. Seeing some of the material for the second time will be a definite "time windfall" which you can use for studying other subjects like human anatomy. You may also want to use that extra time for some other extremely important things—exercise or sleep.

Non-Science Majors

All of the previous recommendations regarding the opportunity to take upper division biology courses also applies to non-science majors. In scheduling these classes, these premedical students (non-science majors) may have certain advantages. First, non-science majors would not be forced to take more than two science courses in any semester. Most upper division biology courses (*e.g.* physiology, histology/embryology, genetics, and anatomy—invertebrate or gross anatomy) only require introductory college biology as a prerequisite. Taking biochemistry usually requires only two courses: introductory college chemistry (inorganic and organic) and biology.

As a non-science major, taking an upper division level biology course(s) will give you the advantage of developing your rote memorization skills that are so essential for surviving the first two years of medical school.

One word of advice when taking these additional biology courses: Don't be intimidated by the course or by the other premedical students taking the class. First, in terms of difficulty, these courses will be no more difficult than any of your other introductory science and mathematics courses. In fact, most students taking these classes find them more refreshing than "trudging through" the material of introductory premedical courses, most of which have nothing to do with the academic content found in medical school. Premedical students find upper division level courses more satisfying because they relate to actual material studied in medical school. These upper level courses can be difficult because of the sheer volume of material which must be comprehended. Memorization skills will be utilized more in these courses than the analytical skills and problem solving abilities needed in chemistry, physics, or calculus.

These classes will also be ones that will be "filled with many other premeds", most of whom will be biology majors. Remember an important golden rule—"Don't be intimidated." Many of the symptoms of "being premed" (discussed in Chapter 6) will be readily diagnosed in some of these classmates. Ignore any so perceived "intimidating tactics" and try to "stay within yourself." Remember the reasons why you are in this course—learning substantive biology material that will help you in medical school. Gaining excellent memorization and time-management skills and maintaining or improving your science GPA will also prove to a medical school admissions committee that you have the ability to handle more difficult biology courses. (These upper division biology classes will also be fundamental to the basic science years in medical school.)

Back to the Basics

I have prepared the following checklist of courses as a guideline to help plan your premed courses. (In Chapter 7 I had discussed various approaches to scheduling your coursework):

1. THE "BASIC FOUR" COLLEGE PREMED SCIENCE COURSES (REQUIRED BY THE VAST MAJORITY OF MEDICAL SCHOOLS):

    1. Introductory Chemistry (with lab): one year (*e.g.* two semesters or three trimesters)

    2. Introductory Biology (with lab): one year

    3. Introductory Organic Chemistry (with lab): one year

    4. Introductory Physics (with lab): one year

2. THE ADDITIONAL "TWO NECESSARY COURSES":

1. English (Composition and/or Literature)

2. College Mathematics (Algebra/Trigonometry, Calculus I, Calculus II)

   (A majority of medical schools will require you to take English courses in college. A smaller number of schools will require either basic college math—algebra/trigonometry or usually calculus I and/or calculus II).

If the areas of "English" and "math" are not required by particular medical schools, they will certainly be listed as courses that are "highly recommended." (Translation: Whether or not these courses are required, it is a good idea to take them in these subject areas.) Most undergraduate institutions recognize the need to take courses in these disciplines and have them either as a "liberal arts requirement" or a "core course" requirement for graduation. In summary, in order to be recognized as "educated men and women who graduate college and who will leave their mark on society,"—it probably makes sense to take some English and math. This same approach in formulating general graduation requirements may also apply to courses in the humanities, social sciences, and behavioral sciences (*e.g.* psychology). Some colleges may also require courses in theology and/or philosophy to graduate.

Keeping this in mind, a small number of medical schools will require you to take one or two semesters of coursework in one or more of these previously mentioned areas (humanities, social sciences, behavioral sciences) to qualify for admission. Whatever a medical school requires or "highly recommends" for subjects outside the science and math areas, remember— DON'T PANIC!; unless your undergraduate school has "no structured graduation requirements" (Translation: Fulfill your major's requirements and then take "whatever other courses you please." These undergraduate schools, however, would be in a distinct minority), you will take courses in the humanities, social sciences, and behavioral sciences. As you can see, these outside course requirements will be fulfilled as part of your graduation requirement. Course selection in these areas will also serve to make you a "well-rounded" and "liberally educated" college student. Keeping this in mind, you want to select these courses carefully; not only do you want to do well academically in these courses, but you want to learn subject matter THAT GENUINELY INTERESTS YOU!

You should also be aware of two other academic options that are offered by many schools: Bachelor of Science degrees and honors programs. To conclude this chapter, both of these options are discussed below.

Bachelor of Science (B.S.) Option

Many college and university science departments will offer a Bachelor of Science (B.S.) option for the student. The Bachelor of Science curriculum is more rigorous than that of the

Bachelor of Arts (B.A.) program—there will be many more additional credit hours required within the major and collateral departments (*e.g.* additional courses in math and chemistry for biology Bachelor of Science majors). Elective credit hours within the major are usually more restrictive because of the additional requirements of the Bachelor of Science program. Because of the high demands of this type of major, students need to start planning their course schedules early in their academic program. The course load usually requires many semesters with three science/ math classes. Because of the rigorous schedule, some students will take summer courses and/or extend their program beyond the four years.

Bachelor of science program requirements are usually specific to each school and must be carefully evaluated before choosing the college/major of your choice.

Honors Programs

Many colleges/universities also offer honors programs. An appropriate GPA will need to be maintained and usually involves independent study courses, research, and /or a senior thesis. Additional coursework in the major (*e.g.* upper level courses or seminars) may also be required. Some programs even allow their students to design their own academic/interdisciplinary major.

9

Premedical Advisors

Just as there is a wide variety of colleges and majors, so it is the same with types of pre-medical advisory departments. In providing guidance to premedical students, there is a gamut of counseling systems that ultimately provide this service. The following listing (along with descriptions) illustrates some of the usual ways in which premedical advice is provided:

1. Premedical Advisory Department, Professor or Administration Official

    Depending on the size of the school, the amount of funding and the number of pre-medical students, one or more advisors are hired from within the academic/administrative ranks of the college/university. Many times these advisors are "paid volunteer" positions; what this means is that a professor (usually with a background in either the biological or physical sciences) who is already teaching courses within the school seeks this job as an additional position or as an extra source of income. The professor (assistant/associate/or full professor) usually has a masters or doctorate (usually a Ph.D.) in his/her academic specialty (many times this is in the biological sciences or physical sciences, such as chemistry or physics). Sometimes the advisor(s) may also have an additional degree in educational counseling and/or a resumé that includes past experience in career counseling.

2. Premedical Advisory Department, "Professional Advisors"

    These positions differ from the first category in that those hired for this position are "full-time" counselors. In the first category, advisors are hired as "part-time." Most "paid volunteer" premed advisors, however, realize that their "part-time" paid position is really a second full-time job with regard to dedication and time commitment. As a premedical student, it is important to seek out those advisors who treat the job as "full-time" and who genuinely care about the students' medical school prospects. (Most premedical advisors do fit into this "commitment category.")

    In the "professional advisory" category, some of these advisors may also teach part-time or be responsible for other programs (besides the premed program), such as student volunteer programs, summer job placement, etc. These advisors may not have a thorough academic background in science but specialize in what they do best—"counseling." They have become thoroughly familiar with the premed curriculum and the medical school application process.

3. Premedical Advisory Committee/Premedical Councils/Professional Health Committee.

These committees include a group of advisors (from either category one or two above or both) who may be individually assigned to a student early in his/her college career and followed through the admissions process. That advisor then writes the student's premed advisory committee letter for medical school. (Note: These committees may also include faculty from non-science departments [*e.g.* English, History, etc.]).

A committee such as this may also interview the students before applying and then review their resumés, academic record, and MCAT scores. One advisor may then be assigned to write the composite letter for the committee on behalf of the student. (Note: If there is an "advisory committee," ask if the committee serves as a "screening committee.") When "screening" is done, it is possible that a student may receive "negative news" that he/she should not apply to medical school based on credentials. This news, however, should "not dissuade" the prospective applicant; the student must ultimately decide whether or not he/she wants to apply—that may have to include one or more applications to a foreign medical school or waiting another year or two to apply. (*e.g.* additional coursework, improving one's GPA and /or MCAT scores)

4. M.D. Advisors

This is a rare occurrence as an undergraduate but consider yourself very fortunate if you are able to get such an advisor. This type of advisor has "truly been through it all." These advisors are able to provide counseling based on personal experience and can give you that extra insight into life as a medical student and as a doctor.

The job responsibilities and duties of the premedical advisory department are numerous. As you review the list on the next page, it will be important for you to identify the strengths and weaknesses in your own college's advisory department. Some schools will exhibit a "stellar performance" in being able to adequately cover all of the enumerated responsibilities. Other colleges will be able to carry out many of them, while others for various reasons (usually funding) will be able to cover only a few.

If there are any weaknesses in the advisory process, the student will still be able to make up for them: You can succeed in overcoming any of these shortcomings by showing INITIATIVE and DISCIPLINE in finding your own sources of information.

DUTIES AND RESPONSIBILITIES OF PREMEDICAL ADVISORS

1. Advisors should help students on decisions about their premedical course selection/scheduling. The idea of "course strategy" should not be taken lightly. Course selection can "make or break" a premedical student's career (especially in the freshman or sophomore years). This individual advice can occur under a variety of circumstances. The following examples help illustrate how an individual's course selection may vary, depending on who the "advisee" is—

   • Advice can be given during orientation to those who declare themselves premed. Follow-up would occur each semester.

   • A sophomore, junior, or senior with little or no science background decides to become "premed."

   • A "switch in career decision": A college graduate or graduate student decides to go to medical school.

   • An adult student who has been away from a full-time school schedule decides to become "premed."

2. Choosing a major (science vs. non-science; other decisions such as "double majors" or a major/minor).

3. Decisions about repeating coursework or taking summer courses.

4. Writing the Premedical Advisory Letter of Recommendation to medical school.

5. Providing references that provide valuable information to medical school applicants; examples include:

   • "The Advisor" (A newsletter written for premedical advisors.)

   • The "Journal of Medical Education" (Gives an annual profile of the year's successful medical school applicants including their GPAs and MCAT scores.)

   • Journal of the American Medical Association (An annual issue on medical education.)

6. Student meetings (individual or group) to discuss such various topics as summer jobs, extracurricular activities, volunteer work, jobs and volunteer activities in health care fields, and MCAT preparation strategy.

7. Guidance regarding the application process itself. (The applicant must stay attuned to the numerous deadlines involved.)

8. Discussion of writing an appropriate personal essay for admission (*e.g.* what attributes and experiences one should focus on in the essay).

9. Information on undergraduate and medical school scholarships.

10. Research opportunities during the academic year or the summer.

11. Development of a "mentor" program. Some advisors may help make arrangements for the student to "shadow a doctor" while seeing patients in the hospital or in the office. (Note: Some undergraduate schools have very strong alumni associations which have strong working relationships with their students; during vacation periods, some alumni agree to let a student(s) "shadow" them during their professional workday. These opportunities may include a variety of areas such as engineering, law, medicine, business management, finance, etc. You should see if there is such an arrangement at your school and ask for the physician list. If there is no formal arrangement, take the INITIATIVE and CONTACT an alumnus/a who practices in an area of medicine that might interest you.)

The areas of medicine that provide both excellent patient contact and a good idea of "what doctors do" include primary care specialties like internal medicine, family practice, pediatrics, or obstetrics and gynecology. Working with a doctor in one of these areas will give you an excellent overview of medicine as a professional career.

12. Information on individual medical schools (*e.g.* school catalogs, sample applications and deadlines, etc.).

13. MCAT information (dates of tests, distribution of MCAT application materials).

14. Maintaining a library of relevant premedical and medical school information.

15. Organization of premed clubs.

16. Bringing in appropriate speakers (*e.g.* physicians, a medical school admissions committee member, etc.).

17. Conducting mock medical school interviews.

18. Compiling statistics (*e.g.* GPAs, MCAT scores) on your college's successful and unsuccessful applicants.

19. Strategies when an applicant is placed on one or more "waiting lists."

20. Strategies for re-applicants.

What Happens if You Encounter a Non-Ideal Advisor/Advisee Situation

As with any process that necessitates the input of various personalities, "no system is perfect because we as humans are not perfect." The premedical advisory process sometimes will show this—there may be personality conflicts between the advisor and the advisee. These conflicts usually occur in only a very small minority of cases; if it affects you, however, that situation is just one too many.

If a problem does arise with an advisor/advisee situation, you should keep in mind two overriding, guiding principles:

1. You are not bound to that one premedical advisor. If it is necessary, you may need to change advisors.

2. Take the INITIATIVE and find out information for yourself if it is not forthcoming from the advisor's office. This book can also serve as an excellent secondary resource because it contains both "pearls of advice" and also detailed information on how to take yourself through the sometimes confusing maze of your premedical years.

Remember that premedical advisors do their best in looking out for the medical school applicant's interest. As previously stated, most premed advisors are doing "full-time work" at "part-time" pay. Their MAIN INTERESTS are those of their premedical advisees. There are, however, some cases where the personality conflicts can potentially affect the applicant's candidacy for medical school admission. Personality conflicts can occur in any type of relationship and that of the premedical advisor-advisee is no different. There are a few premedical advisor personality types that you need to be "aware of":

1. The Premedical "Dissuader"

This type of advisor may seem to be in the "opposite corner"—"Do you really want to go to medical school? Why do you want to go anyway?" . . . "I mean the cost, time, commitment, emotional, and physical drain may just be too much."

2. The "Indifferent" Advisor

This type of advisor does not have his/her heart into the work of premedical advising. Though not as vociferous as the "dissuader," this type of advisor can be anxiety provoking to many medical school applicants: "Where is this advisor coming from?" . . . "What kind of letter will be written for me?" This type of advisor usually gets the job done but the applicant needs to take the initiative early in the application process to make sure an acceptable preadvisory recommendation letter is sent to the medical school.

3. The "Screener"

This type of advisor sometimes has a similar view of medicine as the "dissuader"; also, "average premed students" and those "on the borderline" may hurt the undergraduate school's premed reputation in terms of percentage of accepted medical school applicants.

If misunderstandings occur or tension develops in the advisor-advisee relationship, the premedical student must also take a careful look to see if he/she is the source of the conflict. Advisors are keenly aware of those students who are "acutely affected by the negative signs and symptoms of being premed." These are the students who are known as "grade grubbers," the ones who seek success "at any cost." The problem with some of the students is that their behavior becomes outwardly anxiety provoking and affects those around them. At the least, their personalities are viewed as "disagreeable" and at the worst, they can be seen as "very obnoxious." Students can invoke a negative reaction from others just because of "how they carry on." My advice to those who exhibit these negative premed symptoms is to "TONE IT DOWN!" (It is obvious that hard work and discipline are necessary to achieve your medical school and career goals. Medicine, however, is also about good communication skills and working with a large variety of people and personalities.) The "negative behaviors" of being premed should be avoided because they can be self-defeating; not only can extreme anxiety states harm oneself physically and emotionally, they can also cause others to separate themselves from you. . . . Remember, being an "isolated, anxiety ridden and anxiety provoking" student is not a good way to go through your premedical years!

10
Medical School Selection Factors

Obtaining a position in a first year medical school class has always been a competitive process. What makes it even more challenging today is that it is becoming even more difficult to gain admission! The number of applications has been rising and nearly two out of three applicants will not be admitted. Medical schools are aware of both this acute competition and the need to admit an outstanding first year class. Admission committees will first look at the following areas to see if the applicant is competitive for admission: academic ability and aptitude to successfully complete the medical school coursework; motivation and commitment to a career in medicine; and personal characteristics and qualities that show that the applicant will be a good and compassionate physician. It should also be noted that medical schools will list a variety of selection factors that are important for admitting a class that will help fulfill the school's "goal/mission" in providing quality medical care.

Keeping these principles in mind, it is important to look at the most important factors that can affect an admission decision:

- Objective Academic Criteria
  Grade point average (GPA)
  Science grade point average (SGPA)
  MCAT Scores

- Interviews

- Letters of Recommendation

- Personal Essay

- Motivation and Commitment to a Career as a Physician

- Personal Qualities and Characteristics

- Basic Knowledge About a Medical Career and Issues in Health Care

- Research Experience (if applicable)

- Achievements and Activities
  e.g. Honors and awards   Volunteer Work
        Extracurricular activities   Employment

- Other Factors (*e.g.* state resident)

The next section discusses additional details about many of these factors and highlights the areas which the applicant must understand in the selection process. At the end of this chapter is a list of various opportunities (*e.g.* health care related experience, volunteer work, research, social service, public policy, etc.) that aspiring medical school applicants should find both interesting and worthwhile.

Overview of Some of the Selection Factors

1. Schools want to make sure that their students have the academic ability to "make it through the rigors" of the medical curriculum. This aspect becomes readily apparent as medical students are faced with numerous basic medical science courses during their first two years. GPAs (especially science grade point average) and MCAT scores are very important objective criteria which can help show the candidate's academic achievements and aptitude.

2. In general, medical schools like to see GPAs ranging from a "B" to an "A". Applicants need, however, to know the "specifics"— medical schools will usually publish (e.g. brochure, pamphlet, etc.) grade point averages (cumulative and science) along with average MCAT scores. (Some medical schools may also provide the range of MCAT scores and grade point averages.) There are many medical schools that will have averages of 8-9 or 9-10 on each of the three numerically scored MCAT subsections; other schools will have averages (double-digit, *e.g.* 10-11) that are even higher. Average GPAs are usually from 3.4 to 3.7 (with many in the 3.5 to 3.6 range) for most medical schools. These are again only averages — other factors outside those objective criteria (GPAs and MCATs) will also be important in an admissions decision.

3. Letters of recommendation will also be key factors in the evaluation of your academic abilities. The most helpful letters of recommendation will also be able to discuss your personal attributes and qualities.

4. Your personal essay will also be helpful to an admissions committee. Your life experiences, personal qualities, and the decision to become a physician (along with other appropriate essay themes) will all contribute to a better understanding of why you will be an asset to the medical profession. (For additional information, see Chapter 13, "Letters of Recommendation/ Your Personal Essay".)

5. The medical school interview helps evaluate a number of personal qualities, characteristics,

and skills (*e.g.* communication ability, interpersonal skills, etc.). A comprehensive list of the factors that may be evaluated in a medical school interview are included in Chapter 14, "Interviewing: The Time to Shine".

6. An admissions committee will also look at the candidate's motivation and commitment to become a physician. Evidence of these important factors may include one or more of the following: exposure to clinical medicine (*e.g.* hospital work, physician preceptorships, health care and social service volunteer activities, etc.), having a good understanding of basic health care issues, or participating in a research project.

7. Depending on an applicant's interests, research experience can show evidence of one's commitment and motivation for a medical career. If you are genuinely interested in research and are considering this as a full-time (or even part-time) career, then you should begin to look for these opportunities as an undergraduate. (This is very important if you want to apply to M.D./Ph.D. programs.)

8. There are numerous qualities (*e.g.* compassion, perseverance, leadership ability, being conscientious, self-motivated, etc.) that will help make you a good applicant and physician. Chapters 6 ("Signs and Symptoms of Being Premed: Accentuating the Positive and Avoiding the Negative") and 14 (Interviewing: "The Time to Shine") provide COMPRE-HENSIVE LISTS of exemplary attributes and characteristics. As an applicant, you should be aware of your positive qualities and work to strengthen them. (This same advice also applies to your "weak areas".) Personal growth and development can sometimes take a number of years; you need to be aware of both your strengths and weaknesses so that you can work to achieve your potential as both a person and medical professional. Admission committees need to learn about the "whole person" and will look at the sources (*e.g.* letters of recommendations, personal essays, and interviews) that can provide the insight into the applicant's personal attributes.

A list of various opportunities which include health care related experiences and research activities can be found at the end of this chapter. It should be noted that students can also find similar experiences in their local area; for example, many hospitals have offices which are responsible for "volunteer activities". There may also be other departments in the hospital which may be able to help you set up a preceptorship with a physician. If you are interested in research, many local colleges have science departments that are actively involved in studies covering the biological and physical sciences or an area of medicine. Other excellent resources for research opportunities include any medical schools in your area or a hospital that has residency training programs.

The list at the end of this chapter provides numerous examples of opportunities which are available to college students. (Those programs which have positions available for high school students are also included.) These activities include some of the following areas: research (medical related; biology/life sciences; physical sciences [*e.g.* chemistry and physics]; pharmaceutical company research, etc.), public service, government policy, and medically related externship/internship programs. The student should inquire early in the academic year about these programs because there are a number of factors (*e.g.* funding for the program, application deadlines, prerequisite coursework, stipends, housing/travel allowances, and type of position [paid/volunteer/part-time/full-time]) which can change or be affected in any given year; also be aware that while most of these are summer programs, there also some opportunities that are available during other times of the year.

As to research opportunities, it is important to remember that those programs seek candidates who are GENUINELY INTERESTED AND CURIOUS ABOUT BOTH SCIENTIFIC METHODS AND INVESTIGATION. (Your major, science course background, grades, and letters of recommendation will also be important in obtaining one of these positions.) Funding for these programs may come from a variety of sources: the universities/colleges themselves, government grants, foundations, etc. The funding may sometimes be directed toward programs which have students who may want to have full-time professional research careers. Other programs realize that a student's decision about "going into research" can be difficult without providing some initial exposure to such a career; again, it is important that the student have an "independent and genuine" interest in research. (Many research program directors/committees are adept in separating out the students who are focusing their efforts on "resumé building" from those students who show an avid interest for research.)

Examples of Student Activities and Opportunities

High School Science Research Project Competition

Westinghouse Science Talent Search
Science Service Inc.
1719 N Street, NW
Washington, DC 20036
(202) 785-2255

High School Science Essay Program

The Dupont Challenge
Science Essay Awards Program
Administrative Offices
General Learning Communications
900 Skokie Boulevard, Suite 200
Northbrook, IL 60062-4028
(847) 205-3000
(847) 564-8197 (FAX)
- Grades 7-12.
- An essay about a technological or scientific development, theory, or event (700-1000 words).

Medically Related Research

American Heart Association
- Contact your state affiliate; at the present time, there are no research internship programs at the National Center.
- Cardiovascular research programs: Present high school programs (state affiliates): Hawaii, Nebraska, Washington Present college programs (state affiliates): California, Georgia, Nebraska, Ohio, West Virginia, Oregon.

The Office of Grants Management
Cystic Fibrosis Foundation
6931 Arlington Road
Bethesda, MD 20814
(800) Fight-CF or
(301) 951-4422
(301) i951-6378 (FAX)

- On-going program (applications accepted throughout the year).
- Must be entering a doctoral program (includes M.D. or M.D./Ph.D.), therefore, college juniors/seniors may apply.
- Must do research with a faculty sponsor on a project related to cystic fibrosis.
- If a grant is awarded, students may apply for a subsequent year.
- Previous research experience is not a requirement.

Emory University
1399 Oxford Road
Hughes Science Initiative
Atlanta, GA 30322
(404) 727-4272

Hugh Edmondson Fellowship
University of California, Davis
Medical Center
Department of Pathology
Education Office
4625 Second Avenue
Sacramento, CA 95817
(916) 734-0231

- Variety of research experiences offered (hematology, cancer research, immunology, anatomic pathology, toxicology, etc.).
- Supplemental lectures.
- College undergraduates and graduating high school seniors are eligible to apply.

Summer Student Program
Training and Education Office
The Jackson Laboratory
600 Main Street
Bar Harbor, ME 04609-1500
(207) 288-6250

Myasthenia Gravis Foundation Research Fellowship
Myasthenia Gravis Foundation of America
222 S. Riverside Plaza, Suite 1540
Chicago, IL 60606
(800) 541-5454 or
(312) 258-0522
(312) 258-0461 (FAX)

- Pre-med students eligible. Research must be done under the supervision of a preceptor.

NIH Intramural Student Training Programs
National Institutes of Health
Office of Education
Building 10, Room 1C129
10 Center Drive, MSC 1158
Bethesda, MD 20892-1158
(301) 496-2427
(301) 402-0483 (FAX)

Program Types:
1. College
    1) Summer Internship Program in
       Biomedical Research.
    2) Undergraduate Scholarship Program.
2. Postbaccalaureate
    Predoctoral Intramural Research Training
    Award (recent college graduates planning
    to apply to graduate or professional
    school).
3. Graduate
    1) Summer Internship Program in
       Biomedical Research.
    2) Intern or year-off Intramural Research
       Training Award (for students in doctor-
       al programs).
    3) Predoctoral Intramural Research
       Training Award (for students in doctoral
       programs).
    4) NIH/George Washington University
       Graduate Program in Genetics.
4. Medical and Dental School
    A variety of programs for summer
    research, year-off research experience, or
    clinical electives.

NINDS Summer Program in the
    Neurosciences Office
National Institutes of Health
Building 31, Room 8A19
Bethesda, MD 20892
(301) 496-5332

NINDS: National Institute of Neurological
    Disorders and Stroke
• Training in neuroscience research.
• Lectures and seminars.
• High school (at least 16 years of age),
  undergraduate, graduate, and medical
  students are eligible to apply.

Summer Science Program
Department of Pediatrics
University of Arkansas for Medical Sciences
800 Marshall Street, Mail Slot 512
Little Rock, AR 72202-3591
(501) 320-1847
(501) 320-3551

• Students are assigned to faculty members
  who are working on a research project
  involving children's health.
• Students must have completed at least two
  years of college.

Roswell Park Cancer Institute
ATTN: Summer Research Participation
    Program
Elm and Carlton Streets
Buffalo, NY 14263
(716) 845-2300

• Program for high school juniors.
• Program for college juniors.

Medical Toxicology

Student Summer Research Internships
Society of Toxicology
1767 Business Center Drive, Suite 302
Reston, VA 20190-5332
(703) 438-3115
(703) 438-3113 (FAX)

- Eligibility: depends on geographic internship location — usually at least two to three years of college.
- Science background: depends on project/geographic location.

Internships/Medical Related

Flying Doctors of America
1951 Airport Road
Dekalb-Peachtree Airport
Atlanta, GA 30341
(770) 451-3068
(770) 457-6302 (FAX)

- Medical missions to Mexico, South and Central America, the Dominican Republic, India, and Thailand.
- College self-funded volunteers are welcome to apply. Student volunteers are encouraged to raise sponsorship funds from businesses/church or civic groups/individuals/professionals (e.g. physicians, pharmacists, etc.).

Frontier Nursing Service
Courier Program
PO Box 4
Wendover, KY 41775
(606) 672-2317
(606) 672-3022 (FAX)

- Must be at least 18 years old, have a driver's license, and provide own vehicle (mileage reimbursement).
- Delivery of supplies to clinics, administrative office help, and opportunities to accompany health professionals.
- Unique opportunity in rural health care delivery.
- Volunteer program; minimum two month commitment.

Institute for Mental Health Initiatives
ATTN: Internship Programs
4545 42nd Street, NW
Suite 311
Washington, DC 20016
(202) 364-7111
(202) 363-3891 (FAX)

- January, spring or fall semesters, or summer internship.

Summer Mental Health Internship Program
Foundation for Contemporary Mental Health
2112 F Street, NW, Suite 404
Washington, DC 20037
(202) 296-7100
(202) 296-5455

- Must have completed three years of college.
- Interested in a career in mental health.
- Clinical duties in either a psychiatric inpatient hospital or an outpatient day hospital program.
- Facilities in Washington, DC; Bethesda, MD; and Falls Church, VA.
- Volunteer program.

Internships/Medical Ethics

The Hastings Center
Student Intern Program
Garrison, NY 10524-5555
(914) 424-4040
(914) 424-4545

- Volunteer internships.
- Interns choose their own topic.
- Supervision provided by a specific mentor (staff member at the Hastings Center).
- Participants can attend workshops, discussions, and conferences at the center during their stay.
- Ideal internship times: September through June, typically lasting from two to six weeks.

Pharmaceutical Company Internships

American Home Products Corporation
Corporate Human Resources
ATTN: Student Internship
5 Giralda Farms
Madison, NJ 07940

Bristol-Myers Squibb Company
Human Resources Division
ATTN: Summer Internships
345 Park Avenue
New York, NY 10154-0037
(212) 546-4000

Merck and Co., Inc.
Office of College Relations
ATTN: Summer Internships
One Merck Drive
PO Box 100
U-SUMMCOI
Whitehouse Station, NJ 08889

Procter and Gamble (TN-4)
Recruiting Services Center
ATTN: Summer Internships
PO Box 599
Cincinnati, OH 45201-0599

Wyeth-Ayerst Research
ATTN: Summer Internships
PO Box 7886
Philadelphia, PA 19101
(610) 341-2599
(610) 989-4885 (FAX)

Research
Biological Sciences/Life Sciences

Boston University
Department of Biology
Summer Research in Ecology,
Endocrinology, and Molecular Biology
Boston, MA 02215
(617) 353-2432

Duquesne University
Department of Biological Sciences
Undergraduate Research in Biological
    Sciences
Pittsburgh, PA 15282
(412) 396-5961

Mount Desert Island
Biological Laboratory
PO Box 35
Research Experiences in Marine Physiology
Old Bar Harbor Road
Salsbury Cove, ME 04672
(207) 288-3605

Pepperdine University
Natural Science Division
ATTN: Summer Research Program
24255 Pacific Coast Highway
Malibu, CA 90263-0001

Pomona College
Department of Biology
Summer Research Program in Biology
609 N. College Avenue
Claremont, CA 91711-6339
(909) 607-2993

Washington University
School of Medicine
Department of Anatomy and Neurobiology
660 S. Euclid Avenue
Campus Box 8108
St. Louis, MO 63110
(314) 362-3641

* Summer undergraduate research program
in developmental biology.

Wellesley College
Department of Biological Sciences
Research Program in Biological Chemistry
and Psychobiology
Wellesley, MA 02181
(617) 283-3068

University of Iowa
Department of Microbiology
Undergraduate Summer Research
in Microbiology
Iowa City, IA 52242
(319) 335-7790

Research
Biochemistry/Molecular Biology

Colorado State University
Research Experience for Undergraduates
Program
Department of Biochemistry and Molecular
Biology
Fort Collins, CO 80523-1870
(970) 491-6096
(970) 491-0494 (FAX)

Thomas Jefferson University
Department of Biochemistry and
Molecular Biology
ATTN: Undergraduate Research Program
Philadelphia, PA 19107
(215) 503-4733

University of Minnesota-Twin Cities
Department of Biochemistry
ATTN: Summer Research Program
140 Gortner Labs
1479 Gortner Avenue
St. Paul, MN 55108
(612) 625-2275

* Includes research opportunities in the
medical school.

University of Wisconsin-Madison
Department of Bacteriology
1550 Linden Drive
Madison, WI 53706
(608) 262-2914

* Undergraduate research in cellular and
molecular microbiology.

Research

Molecular Biology/Biomedical & Life Sciences

Summer Undergraduate Research Program
Cold Spring Harbor Laboratory
PO Box 100
Cold Spring Harbor, NY 11724-2213

* College sophomore or junior with a strong academic background.

Research

Biotechnology

Massachusetts Bay Community College
Department of Biotechnology
Research Program in Biotechnology
50 Oakland Street
Wellesley Hills, MA 02181-5399
(617) 237-1100

Research

Physical Sciences/ Biology/ Engineering/Health Sciences

Summer Research Fellowship Programs
Associated Western Universities, Inc.
4190 South Highland Drive, Suite 211
Salt Lake City, UT 84124
(801) 273-8900
(801) 277-5632 (FAX)

* Approximately sixty federal and industrial facilities participate in this program.
* Entering junior year of college.

Research

Physical Sciences/Physics/Engineering

National Astronomy and Ionosphere Center
Summer Student Program
Office of the Director
Cornell University
Space Sciences Building
Ithaca, NY 14853-6801
(607) 255-3735
(607) 255-8803

Summer Undergraduate
Student Visitor Program
High Altitude Observatory
National Center for Atmospheric Research
PO Box 3000
Boulder, CO 80307-3000

* Strong background in physics.
* Entering senior year.

University Programs
NASA/Goddard Space Flight Center
Mail Code 160
Greenbelt, MD 20771
(301) 286-9690
(301) 286-1610 (FAX)

Research

Chemistry

Summer Undergraduate Research Program
Department of Chemistry
Hunter Chemistry Laboratory
Clemson University
Clemson, SC 29634-1905
(864) 656-4200
(864) 656-6613 (FAX)

* At least two years of undergraduate chemistry.

Summer Undergraduate Research Program
Department of Chemistry
University of Georgia
Athens, GA 30602-2556
(706) 542-1936

- Completion of junior year.

University of Kansas
Summer Undergraduate Research Program
Department of Chemistry
Malott Hall
Lawrence, KS 66045-0046
(913) 864-4693
(913) 864-5396 (FAX)

General Scientific Research

Lab Co-op Student Research Participation
   Program
Education and Training Division
Oak Ridge Institute for Science and
   Education
PO Box 117
Oak Ridge, TN 37831-0117

- Sponsored by the Department of Energy.
- Regional sites.
- Applicant must be a college sophomore,
  junior, or senior.
- Variety of scientific disciplines: biology,
  chemistry, computer science, environmental science, engineering, geology, mathematics and related disciplines.

Social Policy/Public Service

Child Welfare League of America
College Internship Program
440 First Street, NW, Suite 310
Washington, DC 20001-2085

- Availability: fall, spring, and summer.
- Duration: average is three to four months;
  some internships have shorter or longer
  periods.
- Policy areas of the organization are numerous but include the following: adolescent
  pregnancy prevention and parenting,
  adoption, child day care, child protection,
  managed health care, etc.
- Minimal compensation.

Healthy Mothers/Healthy Babies Coalition
409 12th Street, SW, Suite 309
Washington, DC 20024-2188
(202) 863-2458

- Most internships are volunteer positions.
- Limited number of paid positions.
- Fall, spring, and summer positions are
  available.

Internship of Victims of Trauma
ATTN: Internship Program
6801 Market Square Drive
McLean, VA 22101
(703) 847-8456

- Volunteer positions (senior in college).
- This organization is a network of professionals trained in crises intervention,
  emergency services, and treatment of post-
  traumatic stress.

Physicians for Human Rights
100 Boylston Street
Suite 702
Boston, MA 02116
(617) 695-0041
(617) 695-0307 (FAX)

- Volunteer program.
- Internships: fall, spring, and summer.
- Locations: Boston, Chicago, Washington, DC.

Government/Public Policy

The Brookings Institution
ATTN: Student Internship Program
1775 Massachusetts Avenue, NW
Washington, DC 20036-2188
(202) 797-6000
(202) 797-6004

- Public policy issues including health care.
- Executive and legislative branch policy areas.
- Part-time and full-time positions.
- Internship positions are volunteer.
- Spring/summer/fall programs.

The White House
White House Intern Program
Room 98
Washington, DC 20500
(202) 456-2742
(202) 456-5123

- Volunteer positions.
- Sessions: fall, spring, and summer.
- At least 18 years old; interns are primarily college juniors and seniors.

Other

Smithsonian Institution
National Air and Space Museum
Summer Internship Program
Educational Services Department, MRC 305
Washington, DC 20560

11

The Medical College Admissions Test (MCAT)

The Association of American Medical Colleges (AAMC) administers the Medical College Admissions Test (MCAT), a standardized test that consists of three multiple choice sections and two writing samples (essays) written by the test taker. The sections, number of questions, and time allotments are as follows:

SECTION	TOTAL NUMBER OF QUESTIONS	TIME ALLOTMENT (MINUTES)
VERBAL REASONING (VR)	65	85
PHYSICAL SCIENCES (PS)	77	100
WRITING SAMPLE (WS)	2	60
BIOLOGICAL SCIENCES (BS)	77	100

The morning session will consist of the verbal reasoning and the physical sciences sections. You will have a ten minute break between the testing sessions. After those parts are completed, you will have a one hour lunch period before the afternoon session of testing. This afternoon session will consist of the Writing Sample section (two essays), a ten minute break, and then the Biological Sciences section, which will be the last part of the test.

Before the actual exam begins, there will be a testing room admission, identification, and administrative information period, which will usually take approximately one hour. The AAMC states that you should be at the test center no later than 8 a.m. It is an excellent idea to get there by 7:30 a.m. so that you do not feel "rushed" or anxious because you are "running late." This process is very formal—photo IDs will be checked, seat assignments will be made, forms will be filled out. . . . All of this occurs even before you receive your first question booklet. DO NOT GET ANXIOUS over all of this administrative "hustle and bustle"— look at it as a procedure that has to be formally done before you "ace your MCAT." Do not look at this waiting period as a time for anxiety and nervousness to build up but rather a short time period when you put your "TEST FACE ON" (NOT YOUR TENSE FACE ON); you need to be physically, emotionally, and mentally ready now. . . .   Test time has arrived. . . .   Make sure you do the things that help you relax . . . *e.g.* taking a few deep breaths, closing your eyes for a few minutes, going to the lavatory before the test begins. . . .   All of these will help get you "test ready"!

WHAT REALLY DOES THE MCAT "TEST"?

First, the MCAT attempts to test medical school candidates' abilities to think analytically and critically, to solve scientific-oriented problems, and to gain a good understanding of scientific concepts that are all within the framework of the basic premedical requirements. Secondly, the MCAT also assesses abilities outside these basic sciences and encourages students to broaden their educational horizons by taking courses in the social sciences and humanities. By providing "verbal reasoning" and "writing sample" sections on the MCAT, the candidates' abilities to think critically, comprehend, and also communicate well are tested.

Subject topics are not specifically tested in the verbal reasoning section. All of the material that you will need for this section appear in the reading passages of the test. The texts to be evaluated will be taken from the social sciences, humanities, and other natural science disciplines. Learning to read with understanding, to think analytically and critically, and to apply the information from the passages will be the keys to success in mastering the verbal reasoning section. Mastering the above skills will also help you to get a good grade on the written essay section of the test. If you learn to read with understanding and also become a "critical thinker," you should be able to master the communication skills necessary to write an essay that is precise and logical. Make sure your spelling, grammar, and punctuation are also very accurate because penalties in these areas can otherwise hurt a "well thought out" and cohesively written essay.

The MCAT cannot predict what kind of doctor you will eventually become— "integrity," "character," "personal qualities", and medical knowledge really play the major roles here (Never equate an MCAT score with your potential status as a medical professional.). At this "moment in time" in your academic career, an admissions committee will use the MCAT score to evaluate your potential in managing a medical school basic science curriculum. The MCAT tends to be the great "equalizer"—it will "even out" the chances of admission for students from a wide array of educational and academic backgrounds and disciplines. For example, if you have been a "stellar" student in all of your basic premed classes, here will be your opportunity to prove that you have both a true understanding of these courses and a very high motivational level to master large amounts of material in preparation for this test. On the other hand, if you have gotten one or more "C"s, or more "B"s than "A"s, doing well on the MCAT will be your chance to prove that you have "all the right stuff" when it comes to tackling the basic sciences. In other ways, admissions committees use the MCAT as the great "equalizer" in trying to make some "objective sense" out of the numerous different schools, GPAs, majors, and course requirements that come across their desks. They sometimes "attempt" to answer some of these "evasive" questions; for example, is the "B" in organic chemistry at Ivy League school "X" the same as the "A" earned at "average" college "Y"? How do you compare the 3.3 student who goes to a highly competitive premed school with the 3.7 student who attends a school not well known for its premed reputation? How about comparing the 3.2 electrical engineering major with the 3.8 history major? The responses to these questions may or may not seem obvious when it involves the admissions process. Looking at MCAT scores, however, can show the committee the applicant's potential for a rigorous basic science curriculum. Remember to keep things in perspective—the MCAT is not a "medical" knowledge test but rather a "premedical knowledge test." Treat it as the "final exam" in your premedical basic science studies. Though it is a VERY IMPORTANT EXAM, the scores DO NOT TRANSLATE INTO HOW KNOWLEDGEABLE AND COMPASSIONATE YOU WILL BE AS A DOCTOR. . . . That will ultimately be left up to you. . . . At the same time, however, if there were no objective means such as the MCAT, "anyone and everyone" would be applying to medical school. . . . What then?

As to the scheduling of your MCAT, the test should be taken in either the spring (April test date) or summer (August test date) of the year you will be applying to medical school. For undergraduates, most applicants would be finishing their junior year (April exam) or getting ready to start the fall semester of their senior year. If you are a "post-college" applicant, you need to carefully plan your coursework or employment because the test would ordinarily be taken the year before you would actually enter medical school. More students take their initial MCAT in April, which allows their applications to be "complete" earlier in the admissions process. Many medical schools utilize a "rolling admissions process"—they start reviewing applications, interviewing, and accepting students as soon as all of their application materials are complete. When an applicant takes the August test, his/her application file will not be considered complete until the scores are reported. (This usually means that their MCAT scores will not be reported until early fall—late September or early October.)

This decision about scheduling the MCAT is a personal one: "YOU MUST STAY WITHIN YOURSELF"—only you know if you are adequately prepared for the test; you should not register for the test "just to take it." A practice "run through" is absolutely not a good decision; what's more, to take the test just so that you can get a head start on the application process is not a good reason if you are not prepared and your scores suffer as a consequence of your decision. (You will definitely not be ahead. . . . You may not get an interview anyway unless you improve your MCAT scores on the August test.) Some students also fall prey to "premed temptations"—every class member they know who is premed is taking the April test. . . . THEREFORE, I HAVE TO TAKE THE EXAM. . . . Do not give in to that "psychological game". . . . YOU MUST TAKE THE EXAM WHEN YOU KNOW YOU ARE READY. Being well prepared and doing well on the April exam is an ideal situation, but it doesn't work that way for everyone. Delaying the test until August may give you that extra preparation time to boost your confidence. With an exam so comprehensive and demanding, many students feel they will never be absolutely ready for the test; again, don't let the test "psyche you out". . . . You will know for yourself if you put forth THAT HONEST EFFORT. . . . If you can answer "yes," then you are ready to take the exam; if you find your scores are not meeting your expectations, you will realize the areas that need improvement and you can then address these problems. "Not meeting one's potential" tends to be a relative term anyway—there are some students who do very well on the MCAT and are still insistent that they could do better (that becomes an even tougher decision as to repeating the test or not). If your scores present more of a "clear cut" picture (below average scores or "acceptable scores"—but not sufficient for the school(s) you would like to attend), then use your extra time in the summer to prepare for the August exam.

As with most important decisions, there are advantages and disadvantages to weigh before formulating an MCAT study plan. As to the timing of your MCAT, these are some of the major factors to consider:

TAKING THE APRIL EXAM

ADVANTAGES

1. Taking this test will allow your applications to be "fully complete" earlier in the process. Many medical schools have a "rolling admissions process"—you may very well be interviewed earlier and accepted.

2. If you need to repeat the exam, you can take the one offered in August. You should still attempt to have your applications completed so that schools will only have to wait for your new scores.

3. If you are currently taking organic chemistry or physics, that material should be "fresh" in your mind. At the same time, however, there will be topics on the MCAT that will not yet have been covered in your formal course. It will be your responsibility to make sure you independently learn those areas. MCAT preparation books and courses are very helpful in this regard.

DISADVANTAGES

1. All of your premedical science courses may not have been completed (see "Advantage No. 3"; you will have to master this new material independently). AVOID TAKING THE MCAT if you still have to take a full basic science course (*e.g.* you have fulfilled all of your requirements except physics). Wait until you take that course or are in its second semester. Some students have taken the MCAT without the advantage of taking a particular course, but this really is an EXCEPTION. It is not the best approach even if you seem to have a grasp of the area from MCAT preparation materials. You want to be able to give yourself the FULL ADVANTAGE of your coursework. The RISK of getting a LOW SCORE in that area could offset any other higher subtest scores.

2. You could have less study time to concentrate on the MCAT exam. Your time-budgeting and organizational skills will be crucial. . . . This is not the semester to overload yourself with extra science courses or a very difficult course load. Think of MCAT preparation as your own extra course that you will have to budget time for!

TAKING THE AUGUST EXAM

ADVANTAGES

1. This allows you sufficient time to complete all of your premedical science requirements.

2. You can spend the summer preparing for the exam. There will be no other semester courses competing for your time. (Your "mind-frame" should have only one academic priority—the MCAT!)

3. Extra time for studying means using it efficiently. . . . Treat your MCAT preparation as a "summer course in itself." A very large amount of MCAT prep book or course materials could be mastered if you PRIME UP your TIME-BUDGETING and ORGANIZATIONAL SKILLS.

DISADVANTAGES

1. Your application will not be considered "complete" until late September/early October because your MCAT scores need to be returned and reported. Processing your formal application and filing secondary applications will also take additional time.

2. If you do not do well enough on this first exam, you will have to wait another year before you can apply. The next test that would be offered would be the one the following April. If this happens to you, use this time to your ADVANTAGE to ACE THE MCAT the next time around.

Formulating Your MCAT "Study Plan"

Keeping all of these factors in mind, it is ABSOLUTELY NECESSARY to formulate a PLAN for "TACKLING THE MCAT." Realizing some general "study for success" principles should help guide you to reach your potential on the MCAT:

1. You can avoid insurmountable test anxiety by preparing early for the MCAT.

2. Using MCAT preparation books and/or formal preparatory courses can help key your success. It is important to use those PREPARATION MATERIALS THAT ARE RIGHT FOR YOU!

3. Proper preparation methods will make your studying more effective.

4. TEST FAMILIARITY is the KEY to DOING WELL.

5. PRACTICE, PRACTICE, PRACTICE! . . .   Do all the practice questions and problems that you can.

"CRAMMING for the MCAT . . . procrastinating until the last weeks will hinder your ability to comprehend and master voluminous amounts of material. Having a study plan that organizes the topics that could be tested on the MCAT is the first place to begin. The *MCAT Student Manual,* which is published by the AAMC, lists all the topics by subject matter (Biology/Chemistry/Physics) and also discusses the reading, writing, and reasoning and problem-solving skills that will be evaluated. This book also offers sample questions and a practice test. Up-to-date MCAT review books and preparatory courses will also have a complete listing of all topics and will have study material (detailed summaries and outlines) and numerous practice problems and simulated exams. (At the end of this chapter is a comprehensive list of resources that can be used to prepare for the MCAT.)

Avoid "spreading yourself too thin" by buying too many review books at one time or by trying to do a formal MCAT course along with some of these other prep books. It is better to finish and master the preparation materials from a smaller number of good resources than to spend time, money, and effort on a number of resources (books, courses) that you only "half finish"!

There are different preparation time frames that are used when studying for the MCAT. Commercial MCAT preparation books and formal courses will all have their suggested time periods and may vary from a couple of months to a year in advance of the test. If the MCAT review is done properly and efficiently, there will also be the critical time period that covers the weeks and days preceding the exam. These shorter preparation periods will not be the time to cram all hours of the day and night. . . .   It will be a time to do numerous practice problems and to take practice exams under simulated time and testing conditions. Taking simulated exams will also build up your "test-taking endurance"—the actual MCAT can prove to be quite exhausting physically, mentally, and emotionally. Developing your test-taking endurance will help you "be your best on exam day" and should help you reach your test potential.

You need to get adequate sleep during the week of the exam. Staying up all hours of the night in final preparation for the test may prove to be counterproductive on the day of MCAT. In order to maintain your stamina for the exam, you really need to be well rested. If you stay well organized with your MCAT study plan, you will be able to avoid both the late night cram sessions and the overwhelming anxiety that accompanies them. Besides doing simulated exams during that week of the exam, you should also spend at least one to two hours a day going over the topics that have been giving you the most trouble. This extra study time should close any learning gaps for the MCAT and will help boost your confidence for the actual exam.

Your concentrated study sessions and reviews for the MCAT should begin three to four months before the actual exam. MCAT preparation books and review courses are designed so that if you hit the "books hard" during this time period, you will be able to reach your potential on test day. This intense preparation period should involve a combination of studying the individual topics and doing practice problems, questions, and exams. MCAT review books and courses will also have numerous practice reading passages and questions that you can use to prepare for the Verbal Reasoning section. These same preparation materials will also have sufficient material to help you practice for the essay section.

Many students often wonder if they can start preparing for the MCAT in their freshman or sophomore year of college. Simply put. . . . YOU CAN! . . . Doing the "little things" early in your premed career will be of definite help when your year for the MCAT arrives. During the first two years of a premedical program, most students will have taken at least three of the four required premed courses. Those courses are usually: 1) general chemistry, 2) introductory biology, and 3) either organic chemistry or physics. Some students may have completed all four courses. At this early point in your premed career, you can buy one or two MCAT review books and start using them as if you were preparing for the real test. . . . Concentrate on those subjects that you just completed. For example, after your freshman year, you may want to study the general chemistry sections and do practice problems and test questions that involve that area. Studying and understanding the solutions/answer explanations to the questions is an excellent method to master the subject.

You will also be able to identify your weak areas and work to strengthen them. Between your actual college course and review materials, you can transform these weak areas into academic strengths. If you truly come to UNDERSTAND the material, your future reviews for the MCAT will be even more effective. Another great idea is to use the *MCAT Student Manual* and cross reference all of those "problem area" subject topics with the appropriate pages in your textbook. If you do this, you will have instant reference material to review your weak areas. You could even go one step further and cross reference these same areas with your lecture notes!

You could do this type of preparation with all of your basic science courses. An excellent time to "leisurely study" is the summer(s) after the courses were taken. You can also do this during the regular school year by reviewing a few subject topics every week. Remember, in these very early MCAT preparation time periods, you do not have to be overly intense. . . . just CONSISTENT AND PERSISTENT! Your hard work and discipline will pay off when you get those good MCAT scores and an admission letter from medical school!

Doing both the verbal reasoning practice passages and the "writing essay" sections from these MCAT review books will also prepare you well for the actual test and will help develop your reading and writing skills. Many students seem to get very anxious about these sections of the exam because they feel they "really cannot study for these parts". . . . This really is a MISCONCEPTION. . . . YOU CAN PREPARE for these sections by PRACTICING, PRACTICING, PRACTICING. . . . GOOD PREPARATION and FAMILIARITY with these areas of the MCAT produce both CONFIDENCE AND SUCCESS on the actual exam!

The purpose of this chapter is to both inform the student about the MCAT itself and to provide various pearls of advice in preparing for and taking the actual exam. The concluding section of this chapter highlights a number of additional factors to remember about the MCAT:

1. The AAMC, along with its member U.S. medical schools, is responsible for developing the MCAT. Registration materials for the exam are provided by your school's premed advisory department or by telephoning or writing the following address:

    MCAT Program Office
    PO Box 4056
    Iowa City, IA 52243-4056
    (319) 337-1357

2. The Association of American Medical Colleges (AAMC) publishes various books/booklets which are very useful to premedical students. Additional information about AAMC resources are found in the MCAT STUDY/REVIEW RESOURCES section at the very end of this chapter.

    In the next major section of this chapter, there is specific information regarding the content of the MCAT. This information is quoted from some of these AAMC publications (*e.g. The MCAT Student Manual* (1995) and *The MCAT Practice Test I*). Requests regarding all publications from the AAMC may be sent to the Association of American Medical Colleges, Department 66, Washington, DC 20055. The Publication Department's phone number is (202) 828-0416.

3. Registration deadlines ("postmarked") for the exam are usually approximately five weeks before the actual exam. Late registration deadlines usually give the applicant another two weeks to apply for the test, but the registration materials must be received (and not post-marked) by their listed dates. (There is also a late fee charged.) Registration materials for the current test period (April/August) will be available after February 1 (of each year).

4. There are a variety of fees (*e.g.* late registration or changing one's test center) charged in addition to the examination fee ($160 in 1997). For those who are in extreme financial need, an MCAT Fee Reduction Program is available.

5. There will be four separate scores reported for each MCAT that the applicant takes; a score will be reported for each section (Verbal Reasoning/Physical Sciences/Writing Sample/Biological Sciences) of the MCAT. A "letter" score, which ranges for "J" (lowest) to "T" (highest), will be given for your writing sample section. Each of the multiple choice sections (Verbal Reasoning/ Physical Sciences/Biological Sciences) will be scored separately based on a scale from "1" (lowest) to "15" (highest). An "average" score for a section is considered to be "8." Be aware that medical schools will have a great disparity of score

requirements and averages for their matriculating class. Some schools, for example, will have MCAT scores that average "10" or higher on each individual subsection.

6. You do not receive an extra penalty for incorrect answers. A separate "raw score" for each section is based on the total number of correct answers. (Do not leave any questions blank — there is no penalty for "guessing.")

7. The Physical Sciences subsection of the MCAT tests your reasoning/analytical skills in general (inorganic) chemistry and physics. Calculus is not tested on the MCAT; therefore, you will only encounter non-calculus based physics problems. The Biological Sciences subtest will assess similar skills in organic chemistry and biology. Each of these sections (Physical Sciences/Biological Sciences) will have 10 or 11 problem sets (each is approximately 250 words in length) and is followed by 4 to 8 questions. There may also be data/information presented in tables, charts, or graphs.

   There will also be another 15 questions in each science section that are independent from the science problem passages and are also separate from each other. The AAMC stresses the fact that the exam evaluates your knowledge of basic scientific concepts and the ability to solve problems, all within the context of biology, physics, and chemistry (organic and inorganic).

8. The Writing Sample section will have two essays that are separately timed (30 minutes each). The AAMC stresses that the essay topics do not refer to the content of basic sciences (biology, chemistry, or physics), about applying to medical school, or to the decision of medicine as a career choice. Religion or issues that could be viewed as emotionally divisive are also not subjects for the essays; social and cultural issues that are not in the "general experience" of college students are also not tested. The AAMC also points out that the essay topics do not evaluate subject matter knowledge.

   Skills of the test taker that will be assessed include developing a central theme; formulating concepts and ideas around your thesis, and presenting your ideas in both a logical and cohesive manner; your ability to write clearly will also be closely evaluated — correct use of grammar, punctuation, and syntax are all crucial for obtaining a good grade on the essay.

9. The AAMC's 1997 *MCAT Announcement* gives the following sample statement (along with sample responses and how they were graded):

   "No matter how oppressive a government, violent revolution is never justified."

In the MCAT Writing Sample section, you are then asked to EXPLAIN what you think the statement means; to DESCRIBE an instance, example, or specific situation that opposes the viewpoint of the statement; and to DISCUSS the factors that would make you think the statement to be true or false.

Again, DO NOT GET UPTIGHT about this section. Comprehensive MCAT preparatory books and courses all have extensive materials on how to prepare for this section. They will also have numerous sample statements with complete answers and explanations as to what makes an essay "below average," "average," or "outstanding." For additional practice, you may eventually want to do your own extra essays and have a teacher from your college's expository writing department review them.

One final word of advice about the Writing Sample section: It is very important that your PENMANSHIP BE LEGIBLE and that your black ink ballpoint be in good working order — black ink smears would certainly make your essay appear "sloppy" and would not present a good "first impression" to the grader/reader.

You must be very attentive to the directions of each MCAT section before beginning it. This was illustrated, for example, with the Writing Sample section. As with any section of the MCAT, not following the directions could prove quite costly to the test taker.

10. Be aware of the time limitations for each section. This factor turns every long standardized exam into an "endurance test." Familiarity with the type of exam questions, along with focused MCAT preparation, will help you adequately budget your time for each of the sections. Practice, practice, practice. . . . Doing simulated exams under the same time constraints will be one of the most advantageous steps you can take for your "MCAT game plan." Remember to take a watch to the exam. You will not, however, be able to take into the exam room a watch that has an alarm, beeping sound, or a calculator function on it.

11. Students use a variety of reading comprehension methods when reading the passages of the Verbal Reasoning section. Spending time doing practice passages and questions will not only help you become a more effective reader, but it will also boost your confidence for the MCAT.

Some students skim the entire passage and look at the introductory and concluding paragraphs to get a quick idea of the text before they go into a more detailed reading. Some spend time reading the questions first and then read the passages; others start "right in" with the passage, reading it in its entirety, while identifying the major concepts and themes. There is also the technique that involves "active reading"—underlining, boxing or circling major ideas, and writing notations in the margin.

Every student has his/her own techniques for being a successful reader. If you spend sufficient time PRACTICING passages and questions, you should be able to discover the METHOD(S) THAT WORK BEST FOR YOU!

13. Eat a light energizing breakfast (*e.g.* juice, toast, fruit, oatmeal, cereal, or some combination, thereof. . . .DO NOT STUFF YOURSELF!). Remember, you need to energize your brain and not overfeed your gastrointestinal (GI) tract! Stay away from caffeine products. . . . They will only serve to increase anxiety/nervousness and may mean extra trips to the bathroom (and thereby taking away precious MCAT test time!).

   This same advice goes for your lunchtime break. You need to choose good foods in the right amounts. . . . You want to be alert for the afternoon sections, not "dulled" by improper food selections.

14. Do not forget to take extra "No. 2" pencils and two black ballpoint pens (for the writing section). Make sure the pens write smoothly because you don't want to have ink smears on your test paper. Be aware that you are not allowed to bring a calculator for the exam.

15. Give yourself plenty of time the morning of the test. You do not want to "be rushed" and feel panicky for the exam.

16. Make sure you get sufficient sleep the week of the exam. You need to be well rested for the MCAT — an exam that not only tests your knowledge but also your endurance!

MCAT Science Topics/Subject Material for the Verbal Reasoning Section / The Writing Sample

The following information is taken from the Association of American Medical Colleges (AAMC's) *MCAT Student Manual* (1995), pp. 36-44 (Chemistry and Physics Topics for the Physical Sciences Section) and pp. 91-101 (Biological Sciences Topics for the Biological Sciences Section):

MCAT SCIENCE TOPICS

1. Physical Sciences Section

(Note: Organic Chemistry is tested under the Biological Science Topics).

1. Underline{General Chemistry Topics}

    1. Stoichiometry
    2. Electronic Structure and the Periodic Table
    3. Bonding
    4. Phases and Phase Equilibria
    5. Solution Chemistry
    6. Acids and Bases
    7. Thermodynamics and Thermochemistry
    8. Rate Processes in Chemical Reactions: Kinetics and Equilibrium
    9. Electrochemistry

2. Underline{Physics Topics}

    1. Translational Motion
    2. Force and Motion, Gravitation
    3. Equilibrium and Momentum
    4. Work and Energy
    5. Wave Characteristics and Periodic Motion
    6. Sound
    7. Fluids and Solids
    8. Electrostatics and Electromagnetism
    9. Electric Circuits
    10. Light and Geometrical Optics
    11. Atomic and Nuclear Structure

2. Biological Sciences Section

    1. Biology Topics

        1. Molecular Biology
        2. Microbiology
        3. Generalized Eukaryotic Cell
        4. Specialized Eukaryotic Cells and Tissues
        5. Nervous and Endocrine Systems
        6. Circulatory, Lymphatic and Immune Systems
        7. Digestive and Excretory Systems
        8. Muscle and Skeletal Systems
        9. Respiratory and Skin Systems
        10. Reproductive Systems and Development
        11. Genetics and Evolution

2. Organic Chemistry Topics

   1. Biological Molecules
   2. Oxygen-Containing Compounds
   3. Amines
   4. Hydrocarbons
   5. Molecular Structure of Organic Compounds
   6. Separations and Purifications
   7. Use of Spectroscopy in Structural Identification

SUBJECT MATERIAL FOR THE VERBAL REASONING SECTION

According to the AAMC's *MCAT Student Manual* (1995), p. 17, subject material for the passages that are in the Verbal Reasoning Section are drawn from the humanities, social sciences, and the natural sciences (excludes the subjects covered in the Physical and Biological Sciences sections of the MCAT):

1. Humanities passages may discuss:
   - architecture
   - art and art history
   - dance
   - ethics
   - literary criticism
   - music
   - philosophy
   - religion
   - theater

2. Social science passages may come from the fields of:
   - anthropology
   - archaeology
   - business
   - economics
   - government
   - history
   - political science
   - psychology
   - sociology

3. Natural sciences passages may cover:
   - astronomy
   - botany
   - computer science
   - ecology
   - geology
   - meteorology
   - natural history
   - technology

THE WRITING SAMPLE

1. Examples of Writing Sample statements:

    1. "Society is best served by giving people as much freedom as possible." (*MCAT Student Manual* (1995), p. 69).
    2. "A nation's ability to survive is often dependent upon its military strength." (*MCAT Student Manual* (1995), p. 79).
    3. "Price is not necessarily a reflection of value." (*MCAT Practice Test I* (1995), p. 47).
    4. "In politics, good intentions cannot justify bad actions." (*MCAT Practice Test I* (1995), p. 48).

2. The Evaluation of Writing Sample Responses by Trained Readers

    According to the AAMC and the *MCAT Student Manual* (1995), p. 67, the evaluation of the student's writing samples by trained readers are as follows:

    "Two readers will score your first essay, and two different readers will score your second essay. Without seeing the other scores given to your writing, each reader will score your response using a six-point scale. The final score for each essay is a function of the scores assigned by the readers. If an essay receives scores that are more than one point apart, the essay is evaluated by a supervisory third reader who determines the final score." (AAMC, *MCAT Student Manual*, p. 67).

    The summarized descriptions of the "typical characteristics" of papers receiving each score are as follows (AAMC, *MCAT Student Manual,* pp. 67-68):

6: These papers show clarity, depth, and complexity of thought. The treatment of the writing assignment is focused and coherent. Major ideas are substantially developed. A facility with language is evident.

5: These essays show clarity of thought, with some depth or complexity. The treatment of the rhetorical assignment is generally focused and coherent. Major ideas are well developed. A strong control of language is evident.

4: These essays show clarity of thought and may show evidence of depth or complexity. The treatment of the writing assignment is coherent, with some focus. Major ideas are adequately developed. An adequate control of language is evident.

3: These essays show some clarity of thought but may lack complexity. The treatment of the writing assignment is coherent but may not be focused. Major ideas are somewhat developed. While there may be some mechanical errors, some control of language is evident.

2: These essays may show some problems with clarity or complexity of thought. The treatment of the writing assignment may show problems with integration or coherence. Major ideas may be underdeveloped. There may be numerous errors in mechanics, usage, or sentence structure.

1: These essays may demonstrate a lack of understanding of the writing assignment. There may be serious problems with organization. Ideas may not be developed. There may be so many errors in mechanics, usage, or sentence structure that the writer's ideas are difficult to follow.

Numerical scores are then converted to an alphabetical score (low score of J to a high score of T). Descriptions of the writing skills associated with the alphabetical scores are summarized in the *MCAT Practice Test III* (1995), p. 118):

Description of Writing Skills Associated with Writing Sample Alphabetic Scores

J	K	L	M	N	O	P	Q	R	S	T

BELOW AVERAGE

These essays demonstrate a degree of difficulty in discussing the topic and/or responding to the three writing tasks. They may show problems with the mechanics of writing or in addressing the topic at a complex level. The response may not be organized, and ideas may not be integrated. Although the three writing tasks may be addressed, the ideas may be underdeveloped.

AVERAGE

These essays demonstrate a degree of proficiency in discussing the topic and/or responding to the three writing tasks. Few problems in the mechanics of writing are evident, and there is demonstration of control of language. The writing tasks are addressed in a clear, organized, and coherent manner. Ideas are developed to some extent and may show evidence of depth and complexity of thought.

ABOVE AVERAGE

These essays respond to the topic and the three writing tasks in a superior manner. The writing demonstrates a strong control of language. The response is presented in a clear, organized, and coherent fashion. Ideas are well-developed, and the topic is dealt with at a complex level.

MCAT STUDY/REVIEW RESOURCES

1. Association of American Medical Colleges (AAMC)
    Membership and Publication Orders
    2450 N Street, NW
    Washington, DC 20037-1126
    (202)828-0416

    1. AAMC, *MCAT Student Manual* (1995): Specific detailed information about the format and science content of the MCAT. A full length practice test is included.

    2. AAMC, *MCAT Practice Test I* (1995).

    3. AAMC, *MCAT Practice Test II/MCAT Practice Items* (1995): The practice test is a reprint of the 1991 (April) MCAT.

    4. AAMC, *MCAT Practice Test III* (1995): Many sample test questions from the 1994 MCAT.

It will be very important for the student to send for annual updates on the AAMC's publications to see if there are any new released practice exams.

1. *ARCO's MCAT Supercourse, 3rd ed.* New York, NY: Macmillan General Reference, 1996. (This book also includes *ARCO MCAT Sample Exams* which can be purchased separately.)

2. Bosworth, Stefan, et al. *ARCO MCAT Sample Exams*. New York, NY: Macmillan General Reference, 1996.

3. Bresnick, Stephen D. and Bresnick, William H., *Columbia Review MCAT Practice Tests*. Baltimore, Maryland: Williams and Wilkins, 1997.

4. Columbia Review's *Intensive Preparation for the MCAT.* Baltimore, MD: Williams and Wilkins, 1996.

5. Hassan, Aftab S., ed. *The Betz Guide: A Complete Preparation for the MCAT*. Baltimore, MD: Williams and Wilkins, 1997.

6. The Princeton Review. *Flowers and Silver MCAT 1997-1998 Edition*. New York, NY: Random House, Inc., 1996.

7. Research and Education Association (REA). *The Best Test Preparation for the MCAT.* Piscataway, NJ: Research and Education Association, 1995.

8. Rothstein, Rochelle, ed. *MCAT Comprehensive Review.* New York, NY: Kaplan Educational Centers and Simon and Schuster, 1997.

9. Silver, Theodore, M.D. and the Staff of the Princeton Review. *Flowers and Silver Annotated Practice MCATs*. New York, NY: Random House, Inc., 1996.

The following two courses are available nationally. Those studying for the MCAT should contact the following review courses for the nearest test center.

FORMAL MCAT PREPARATORY COURSES

1. Stanley H. Kaplan Educational Center
    810 Seventh Avenue, 26th Floor
    New York, NY 10019
    (800)527-8378 or
    (800)KAP-TEST

2. The Princeton Review
    2315 Broadway, 3rd Floor
    New York, NY 10024-4332
    (800)995-5565

REGIONAL MCAT COURSES

1. The Columbia Review
    220 Madison Avenue
    San Francisco, CA 94134
    (800)300-PREP or
    (415)337-2009

    1. States: California, Washington, Arizona, and Texas (Austin).
    2. Offers a formal home study course.

2. The Berkeley Review
    PO Box 40140
    Berkeley, CA 94704
    (800)622-8827 or
    (510)843-8378

    1. Regional: California.
    2. Offers a formal home study course.

When looking at these courses, many of the following factors should be considered:

1. Review books/materials
2. Sample problem sets
3. Sample tests
4. Classroom lectures
5. Average class size
6. Recorded tapes of lectures/reviews/solutions to problem sets/solutions to sample MCATs
7. Cost
8. Formal lectures/meetings per week
9. In-class simulated MCAT exams
10. Availability of tutoring
11. Length of the course
12. Opportunities to repeat the course or extend the length of the course

REFERENCES

1. The Association of American Medical Colleges (AAMC), *MCAT Announcement,* Washington, DC, 1997 (updated annually).
2. AAMC, *MCAT Practice Test I*, Washington, DC, 1995.
3. AAMC, *MCAT Practice Test III*, Washington, DC, 1995.
4. AAMC, *MCAT Student Manual*, Washington, DC, 1995.

12
The Medical School Application Process

AMCAS and NON-AMCAS SCHOOLS

The American Medical College Application Service (AMCAS) is a centralized application service that is used by students applying to the majority of U.S. allopathic (M.D.) medical schools (for the 1997-1998 application year, only 15 are non-AMCAS schools and require separate applications; a listing of non-AMCAS is found at the end of the first section of this chapter). This processing service makes it easier for both the students and medical school during the application year: The AMCAS standardized application form, biographic and academic data, and MCAT scores are sent to the AMCAS participating schools requested by the student. For the non-AMCAS medical schools, you must send their individual application forms along with making arrangements to send your MCAT scores and grade transcripts. There are a number of different types of applications used by these non-AMCAS schools; these applications are individualized to that particular school. Always use that school's individual application; never send a photocopied AMCAS application form—if you do, it will be "bad form."

With the standardized AMCAS application form, the student can apply to as many medical schools as he/she desires but is charged according to a fee schedule. For the 1997-1998 application year, a $50 fee is charged for using the AMCAS service (This also entitles you to one processed application.); a fee schedule is then provided, which is based on the number of designated medical school applications (*e.g.*, $170 for 4 schools, $275 for 8 schools, $450 for 15 schools, etc.). If you submit your AMCAS application (with appropriate fees) and then decide you want to have more applications processed, a second fee schedule (Fee Schedule for Additional Designations) is provided.

The AMCAS paper application form SHOULD BE TYPED. There is now an electronic form of the AMCAS application (AMCAS-E) that helps to accelerate the application process. The software allows for both grade/credit-hour conversions and also has a self-audit for all required data forms. If the student decides to use AMCAS-E, a computer disk (and not paper materials) will be submitted to AMCAS. The student, however, will still be able to print completed copies of the AMCAS forms for one's personal file. The AMCAS-E for Windows software may be downloaded from the Internet Web site at http://www.aamc.org.

There are different ways of obtaining the traditional AMCAS paper application or the electronic form (AMCAS application material is available every April for the following year's entering class):

1. Write or telephone: American Medical College Application Service (AMCAS)
                           Association of American Medical Colleges
                           Section for Student Services
                           2501 M Street, NW, Lbby-26
                           Washington, D.C. 20037-1300
                           Telephone: (202) 828-0600

2. AMCAS application material may also be available from your premed advisor/Health Advisory Committee/Career Advisory Office.

3. Send E-mail requests to amcas @ aamc.org. If you desire the traditional application, enter "amcas-paper"; if you request the electronic version, type "amcas-win." Your preference should be typed in the "subject line."

4. The materials can also be ordered on the AAMC Web Internet Web site at:

    http://www.aamc.org.

Osteopathic medical schools also use an application service: The American Association of Colleges of Osteopathic Medicine Application Service (AACOMAS). For more information or to send for a formal application, telephone or write:

American Association of Colleges of Osteopathic
Medicine Application Service (AACOMAS)
5550 Friendship Blvd., Suite 310
Chevy Chase, MD 20815-7231
Telephone: (301) 968-4190

There is also an electronic form of the AACOMAS application. "AACOMAS by computer (ABC)" can be requested on the Web site at http://www.aacom.org. (Note: It is necessary to have a 386 computer [or higher] with Windows 3.1 or 95. You can order a diskette of the program by telephoning (301) 968-4190.

NON-AMCAS SCHOOLS

It is important to note that as of this copyright publication date, there are 15 non-AMCAS schools. Each has a separate application, and you must provide all the supplementary information separately (*e.g.* official transcripts, official MCAT score reports). There will be separate fees associated with the application itself and the processing of MCAT scores and grade transcripts. A listing of these schools is below:

1. Harvard Medical School

2. Johns Hopkins University School of Medicine

3. University of Missouri (Kansas City) (six-year BS/MD program)

4. New York University School of Medicine

5. University of North Dakota School of Medicine and Health Sciences

6. Brown University School of Medicine

7. Columbia University College of Physicians and Surgeons

8. Baylor College of Medicine

9. Texas A & M University Health Sciences Center College of Medicine

10. Texas Tech University Health Sciences Center School of Medicine

11. Yale University School of Medicine

University of Texas:

12. Southwestern Medical School (Dallas)

13. University of Texas Medical School at Galveston

14. University of Texas - Houston Medical School

15. University of Texas Medical School at San Antonio

Applications to these last four medical schools are made through a separate application service:

University of Texas System Medical and
Dental Application Center
702 Colorado, Suite 620
Austin, TX 78701

Be aware that the list of non-AMCAS schools may change in any given application year. If a medical school is not listed on the AMCAS DESIGNATION FORM, then the school has its own separate application. Be sure to check that list in the AMCAS application during the year you are applying. Your AMCAS application and booklet will provide the appropriate information each year regarding non-AMCAS schools.

The AMCAS Application Form

The application is very detailed and covers a large number of areas and concerns. A THOROUGH READING of the application booklet is ABSOLUTELY NECESSARY to properly complete the AMCAS application.

The following information is necessary to complete the application:

(See Association of American Medical Colleges, *AMCAS® Instruction Booklet for the 1998 Entering Class,* 1997. At the end of this chapter are sample forms which are used with the permission of the AAMC.)

PART I

1. Social Security Number

2. Full Name

3. Permanent Address (may not correspond with the applicant's state of legal residence or preferred mailing address)

4. Permanent Telephone Number (may not correspond with the applicant's preferred telephone number)

5. Parents/Guardian

   - Name
   - Living/Deceased
   - Occupation
   - Legal residence
   - Education/college (highest level)

6. Ages of Siblings

7. Secondary School/High School Name, Address, and Graduation Year

8. All Colleges Attended (undergraduate/graduate/professional school)

   - Chronological order

- Location/dates of attendance/summer school (?)/junior college (?)
- Major/degree granted (or expected); date of degree (If "no degree," put "none"—*e.g.* summer courses or semester(s) spent at one school before transferring.)

9. Post-Secondary Honors/Awards

10. Extracurricular, Community, and Avocational Activities

11. Post-Secondary School Employment History (chronological order; may include part-time, full-time, and/or volunteer work)

PART II

"Personal Comments" (Personal Essay)

The space provided to type is slightly smaller than 8 1/2 inches x 11 inches. This application essay is limited to the one page. Note that Part I items, (No. 9-11) from above, may be continued in this section. The extra lines used for continuing "Part 1 items" will take away from essay space—the applicant is not allowed to submit supplementary type-written pages—the only page space allowed is that which occurs in the formal application.

PART III

Academic Record

This section will give a detailed listing of every course you have attempted in college, graduate school, or another professional school. All of your grades (including, for example, advanced placement, CLEP, audit courses, etc.) and course transactions (*e.g.* "Incomplete," "Repeat," "Withdrawal," etc.) will be your responsibility to fill out accurately. You will have to get copies of official transcripts from every college attended so that all information is accurately recorded. Credit hours and GPAs will also be calculated, using a uniform conversion system used by AMCAS. You must read the instructions carefully so that all course entries and conversions are accurate. For example, some students are on a quarter-hour system and will be able to accurately convert those credit hours to a semester-hour system. Also, some schools do not recognize "+'s" or "-'s" in their grading calculations. A college may only give a 3.0 value for a "B+" grade whereas AMCAS converts this to a 3.3. At the same time, however, if your school gives a 3.0 for a "B-," your AMCAS conversion will be 2.7. To provide uniformity, AMCAS will give numerical values to "+" and "-" grades. What's more, some schools still use numerical grades (*e.g.* 93-100 is an "A"), and using the AMCAS system, these numbers can be converted into an equivalent GPA. As to an applicant's GPA, a science (biology/ chemistry/ physics/math courses) GPA will be calculated for each year along with a non-science GPA. The total GPA for each year (along with your final cumulative GPAs in science and non-science areas) will also be shown on the AMCAS record. If appropriate, any post-baccalaureate courses or graduate courses will also have their separate GPA calculations.

It will be the applicant's responsibility to make sure all MCAT scores and college/graduate transcripts are forwarded to the AMCAS service. Your academic record will be formally reviewed and checked against official transcripts to verify all course designations, grades, and credit hours. A formal AMCAS application will then be sent to each medical school that you designate. Each medical school will not receive a transmittal record listing the other medical schools that you have designated to receive an application. (Simply put, each medical school will not know about your other applications from your AMCAS records.)

AMCAS medical schools have deadlines by which all materials (including application forms and transcripts) must be received (and not merely postmarked) by AMCAS. The application deadlines generally are October 15/November 1/November 15/December 1/and December 15, but each school that you apply to has only one of the above dates. You need to check the AMCAS booklet each year for the deadline categories and the schools listed under each of these dates. It will also be very important to make sure these dates match with those mentioned in any of the materials (brochures, catalogs) that you receive from each medical school.

At the same time, you must be very attentive to meeting all the deadlines of any non-AMCAS schools that you apply to—there is no corresponding application service for them, so you must follow up carefully to make sure all of your application materials get there on time! Your ORGANIZATIONAL SKILLS (DON'T PROCRASTINATE!) will be crucial in making sure all deadlines are met. . . . Missing a deadline, unfortunately, could mean the rejection of even a very well-qualified applicant.

To verify that the AMCAS application has been sent, you will receive a Transmittal Notification Form from AMCAS that will list essential biographical information, college atten-dance record, GPA information, MCAT scores, and a list of medical schools where your appli-cation was sent.

It is important to note the following additional points about AMCAS services:

1. AMCAS is only an application PROCESSING SERVICE. It has nothing to do with the actual admissions decision process.

2. AMCAS is for first-year applications to ALLOPATHIC (M.D.) medical schools. If you are considered an "advanced standing" or a transfer medical student applicant, you should call or write the schools directly. Osteopathic medical schools have their own application pro-cessing service (AACOMAS), which was discussed in this chapter.

3. There is a fee-waiver program (medical school applicants with financial "inability to pay" limitations) that allows qualifying students to apply up to ten AMCAS schools without paying the appropriate service fee.

4. The EARLY DECISION PROGRAM (EDP) has the earliest AMCAS application and transcript receipt deadline (for example, the deadline at AMCAS was August 1, 1997, for the Entering Class of 1998); all other AMCAS schools' deadlines ranged from October 15 - December 15, 1997.

5. Additional Designation Form: An applicant can request that additional AMCAS schools (separate fee schedule) be sent an application after the original school designation form was sent with the AMCAS application.

6. Changes or corrections during the verification process of your AMCAS application can be made by submitting a post-submission change form.

AFTER AMCAS. . . .

Medical schools will review and evaluate your AMCAS application. Some schools may make their "first cut" based on this application and send out their first rejection letters; others may require all/some of their applicants to fill out secondary applications. (Some medical schools will charge additional fees with these secondary applications.) Updated transcripts and/or MCAT scores may also be required before a final decision can be made by the admissions committee.

Letters of recommendation (usually they are part of the "secondary application") should be sent directly to the AMCAS schools. You must meet the individual deadlines and specific requirements; medical schools have their own policies about recommendation letters: *e.g.* two letters from science instructors and one from a teacher in a non-science course. Do not make the mistake of sending these letters to AMCAS—they will send them back to you. What's more, you may miss a medical school's deadline if you don't follow the instructions in the supplementary application materials.

SECONDARY APPLICATIONS

Upon review of your AMCAS application, many schools will send you a "secondary application." The length of these forms may vary from a couple of pages to four or more pages. Pay close attention to the instructions, requirements for additional documents (*e.g.* letters of recommendation, updated transcripts, or your latest MCAT scores), and appropriate deadlines. Letter of recommendation forms may be enclosed along with instructions on who would be appropriate sources for these letters. Again, follow those instructions carefully; if a medical school states that it wants only three letters, do not send them six! Some schools are very strict about these numbers but many give the applicant an option to send additional letters (. . . of course, with number limitations). Every medical school has individualized requirements, but the following list gives an idea of the general categories:

1. College or university faculty from any department

2. A science department faculty member (one or more letters)

3. Premed committee evaluation report/premed advisor letter

4 Letters from those who know you well from community service or from a health care volunteer or health care work experience

5. Letters from employers (usually for candidates who have been out of college several years)

6. Note: Many osteopathic medical schools will require the applicant to obtain a letter from an osteopathic physician.

7. Letter from the person who sponsored or coordinated your research project (if applicable).

The applicant may also be asked to write additional essays or short answers to questions in the secondary application. Some of these essays may be similar to the AMCAS personal essay or may ask you to further discuss your extracurricular activities, hobbies, volunteer, and health care related work (if applicable). Some other schools may ask you to write on a specific topic (*e.g.* health care reform) or write about your motivation to become a physician.

Non-AMCAS schools will, of course, have longer applications (compared to the secondary ones) because they do not accept the uniform AMCAS form. In most instances, you will be typing the same information, but it will appear in slightly different form than the AMCAS application. Again, pay close attention to all of their deadlines because you will be responsible for MCAT score reports and grade transcripts getting to those schools on time. Letters of recommendations will also be sent, so it is essential that you follow the non-AMCAS school's requirements.

OTHER IMPORTANT FACTORS FOR ADMISSION

TECHNICAL STANDARDS

Medical schools will clearly define their technical standards for admission that will encompass a variety of requirements including an applicant's physical, emotional, and psychological well being. Examples of such standards include: abilities to observe and to communicate, sufficient motor skills, behavioral and social attributes, and integrative, intellectual/conceptual and quantitative abilities.

RESIDENCY REQUIREMENTS

Applying to a state university medical school as an out-of-state resident can be very difficult, or in some cases, "insurmountable." There are some state medical schools that consistently fill their classes with 100 percent state residents. There are also many other state schools that consistently admit greater than 90 percent of their class from the state resident applicant pool. (Note: Some schools will not even send information or secondary applications based on your out-of-state residency status. These medical schools usually report that the number of highly qualified residents from their state far exceeds the available number of class positions.) If there is a question about your residency status, you should direct your questions to that particular school. Many state universities will send a residency classification guide or booklet, which will help you determine your residency status for that particular state school.

Also, some state medical schools will accept applications and admit students who are children of alumni from that medical school or state university system. There is no uniformity, however, regarding this policy; it is best to consult directly with the appropriate medical school if this category describes your application status.

IF YOU ARE ACCEPTED . . .

You must carefully review all the medical school's application materials and information as to acceptance procedures. Catalogs, brochures, and pamphlets may be good sources for this information, but many schools inform the accepted applicant directly about the procedures and requirements.

The AAMC has its own recommendations for acceptance procedures. Medical schools usually follow these recommendations as their own, but you need to look at the procedures of each school that accepts you. . . . Be aware of these dates—write them down along with the acceptance deposit fees that are required. You need to follow these directions precisely so that there is no confusion about filling and maintaining that spot in the first-year class.

Some of the highlights of the AAMC's Recommendations Concerning Medical School Acceptance Procedures for First Year Entering Students are as follows (AAMC's *Instruction Booklet for the 1998 Entering Class*, p. 23):

1. Medical schools are asked not to notify before October 15 any applicant who has been accepted.

2. Any time before May 15, an accepted applicant should be allowed two weeks to accept that school's offer of admission

3. After this date (May 15), medical schools could require the accepted applicant to reply in less than two weeks. The accepted applicant could then be required to pay a deposit and/or file a "statement of intent." (If the applicant is later accepted by a medical school that he/she prefers, the applicant should have the freedom to withdraw that acceptance from the original school.)

4. After May 15, medical schools are allowed to make rules for accepted applicants who "hold"

places in more than one medical school. (If a medical school has its first official class day before August 1, it can begin to ask for accepted application decisions before May 15 [but not before April 15]).

5. An acceptance deposit should not be more than $100 and should be refundable until May 15. If the student attends that medical school, it is encouraged that the amount be credited towards tuition. It is possible that a school could keep that fee as a "late withdrawal fee" if the accepted applicant does not attend the school.

(NOTE: Most of these recommendations do not apply to applicants accepted through the Early Decision Program. These students have already agreed to attend a certain medical school if accepted through the Early Decision Program.)

These are some of the recommendations that highlight the acceptance process. They are promulgated in order to provide uniformity and efficiency to a process that involves "thousands of acceptances"! The goals are not only to avoid administrative and bureaucratic confusion but also to give every applicant a fair opportunity to either attend a medical school or go to the medical school of his/her choice.

Finally, in making your decision, you must CHOOSE THE MEDICAL SCHOOL THAT IS RIGHT FOR YOU! If you receive just one acceptance letter . . . remember, that's all you need, DOCTOR!; otherwise, you should weigh all those factors (*e.g.* financial, educational/clinical advantages, geographical area, "school personality") before you make your choice. Chapters 16 ("Questions You Should Ask About Medical Schools") and 24 ("Financing Your Medical School Education") may help give you additional guidance for your decision.

IF YOU ARE WAIT LISTED. . . .

This can prove to be a very challenging time period for the applicant. If he/she has received no other acceptances, it can even be more difficult. . . but stay OPTIMISTIC! . . . There is still a chance for acceptance. . . . Medical schools will accept applicants from their waiting lists during the spring, summer, orientation week. . . and yes, even after the first class has started.

As seen in the previous section, there are deadline dates that accepted applicants must follow—there are "response time limitations" for students holding a position (one or more acceptances) in more than one school. Medical school admission committees have to make sure that they receive a response from each accepted applicant; only after responses are received and a determination that openings exist, can a wait-list applicant be considered.

You should also remember to continue to communicate with the school(s) that have placed you on a wait-list(s). . . .Show the school(s) that you are interested but do not "overdo it" with excessive telephone calls and letters. You should make sure, however, that the premedical advisory office knows about your status and that the medical school(s) is informed about any personal updated information (*e.g.* grades, honors and awards, achievements in extracurricular activities or volunteer work, employment activities, etc.)

Information on Individual Medical Schools

Medical school brochures, pamphlets, catalogs, and bulletins are resources for detailing the information about an individual institution. The Association of American Medical Colleges publishes *Medical School Admission Requirements, United States and Canada 1998-1999* (editions are updated annually) and Part II of that book lists individual entries of all medical schools in the United States, Puerto Rico, and Canada. The information about the medical schools is provided directly by them and includes the following entries:

1. General Information
2. Curriculum
3. Requirements for Entrance
4. Selection Factors
5. Financial Aid
6. Information for Minority Students
7. Type of School: Public/Private Institution
8. Application and Acceptance Policies
9. Tuition and Student Fees
10. Information on the Previous Year's First Year's Class

(Number of applicants/interviews [in-state and out-of-state applicants] and new entrants in the first year class.)

Other Unique Application Circumstances

1. EARLY DECISION PROGRAM (EDP)

Over eighty medical schools participate in the Early Decision Program (EDP). The advantage of such a program is that the student knows early in the application year whether or not he/she has been accepted to medical school. If the student is accepted by a medical school which offers an Early Decision Program, he/she must attend that school (an applicant can apply to only one medical school [AMCAS and non-AMCAS schools] under an Early Decision Program).

A student must meet the application deadline of an AMCAS (August 1) or a non-AMCAS school (check the individual school's deadline). Applicants are required to be notified of an acceptance/non-acceptance by October 1. Deadline and notification dates may change in a particular year, so it is important to check for that information during your application year to medical school. If the applicant is not accepted by a medical school under the Early Decision Program, he/she will have adequate time to apply to other medical schools. (NOTE: Some medical schools only offer an Early Decision Program for state residents).

2. APPLICANTS WITHOUT AN IN-STATE MEDICAL SCHOOL

1. WICHE Program (Western Interstate Commission for Higher Education)

Residents of Alaska, Montana, and Wyoming are eligible to apply to a number of medical schools under the Western Interstate Commission for Higher Education (WICHE) Professional Student Exchange Program. If accepted by a participating medical school, the student pays that state's resident tuition (at a public institution) or a reduced tuition at a private school. Such fee agreements regarding tuition exist because the "sender states" pay "support fees" to the participating medical schools to help cover the educational costs. The student must be "certified" by his/her state of residence in order to be eligible as an applicant. This process of certification establishes that an applicant is a resident of the "sending state" and is eligible to apply if adequate state funds are available.

More information can be obtained by contacting the WICHE Professional Student Exchange Program:

Western Interstate Commission for
Higher Education (WICHE)
Professional Student Exchange Program
PO Drawer P
Boulder, CO 80301-9752
(303)541-0214

(NOTE: WICHE will have a list of addresses and telephone numbers of the certifying officers of the participating states).

The list of participating medical schools is as follows:

Participating "sender states": Alaska, Montana, Wyoming.

PARTICIPATING (M.D.) MEDICAL SCHOOLS (WICHE Program)

ARIZONA
University of Arizona College of Medicine

CALIFORNIA
Loma Linda University School of Medicine
Stanford University School of Medicine
University of California, Berkeley/UC San Francisco Joint Medical Program
University of California, Davis, School of Medicine
University of California, Irvine, College of Medicine
University of California, Los Angeles, UCLA School of Medicine
University of California, San Diego, School of Medicine
University of California, San Francisco, School of Medicine
University of Southern California School of Medicine

COLORADO
University of Colorado Health Sciences Center School of Medicine

HAWAII
University of Hawaii John A. Burns School of Medicine

NEVADA
University of Nevada School of Medicine

NEW MEXICO
University of New Mexico School of Medicine

NORTH DAKOTA
University of North Dakota School of Medicine

OREGON
Oregon Health Sciences University School of Medicine

UTAH
University of Utah School of Medicine

OSTEOPATHIC (D.O.) MEDICAL SCHOOL (Participant in the WICHE Program)

Western University of Health Sciences/College of Osteopathic Medicine of the Pacific (Participating states: Alaska, Arizona, Hawaii, Montana, New Mexico, Oregon, Washington, Wyoming)

2. WAMI PROGRAM (Washington, Alaska, Montana, Idaho)

Students from the states of Alaska, Montana, and Idaho spend their first year of medical school at designated universities in their home states. Students then attend the University of Washington for their second year of medical school. More information on this program can be obtained by contacting the University of Washington School of Medicine:

Admissions Office
University of Washington
School of Medicine
Box 356340
Seattle, WA 98195-6340
(206)543-7212

To conclude this chapter, I have enclosed five pages of sample AMCAS® forms. The following forms are used with the permission of the Association of American Medical Colleges and can also be found in the AMCAS® *Instruction Booklet for the 1998 Entering Class,* (pp. 29-32; 36):

1. AMCAS® Application for the 1998 Entering Class (also includes pages for the applicant's personal comments and his/her academic record.)

2. AMCAS® Transmittal Notification page.

1. SSN 028-26-2288	AMCAS® APPLICATION FOR THE 1998 ENTERING CLASS	AMCAS USE ONLY

2A. Last Name ZYLER	2B. First Name Richard	2C. Middle Name Ross	2D. Suffix III

3A. Permanent Address - Street 434 Columbus Avenue, Apt. 2	3B. City (and Province) New Haven	3C. St CT	3D. ZIP/Postal Code 06519 - 1234

3E. County (if in U.S.A.) New Haven	3F. Country (if not U.S.A)	4. Telephone (203) 555-5125

5. PARENTS OR GUARDIAN

Name	Living?		Occupation	Legal Residence	Education/College (highest level)
	Yes	No			
Father Ralph E. Zyler	x		Teacher	Mass.	M.A., Boston Univ.
Mother Edwina Alexander	x		Economist	Calif.	Ph.D., Harvard
Guardian					

6A. Ages of your Brothers 9	6B. Ages of your Sisters	7A. Secondary School - Name William Penn H. S.	7B. City, State (Country if not U.S.A.) Davis, CA	7C. Grad Yr. 1988

8. ALL COLLEGES, GRADUATE AND PROFESSIONAL SCHOOLS ATTENDED (list in chronological order)

Name	Location (City & State)	Dates of Attendance MM/YY to MM/YY	Check if summer only	Check if Jr/Comm College	Major	Degree Granted or Expected (with date)
Sorbonne	Paris, France	6/88 - 8/88	x		French	None
Bennett College	Millbrook, NY	9/88 - 8/89		x	Science	None
Nassau Cmty. Col.	Garden City, NY	9/89 - 6/90		x	Biology	None
Michigan State U.	East Lansing, MI	9/90 - 8/91			Biology	None
EFGH College	Washington, DC	9/91 - 6/92			Biology	B.S. 6/92
St. Mercy Hospital	Duncannon, PA	1/92 - 6/92			Med Tech	None
XY State Univ.	Washington, DC	9/92 - 6/96			Psych	M.A. 6/96
Abcd University	Washington, DC	9/96 - 6/97			Microbiol	None
		-				
		-				

9. Post-Secondary Honors/Awards:

Phi Beta Kappa· Dean's List for three semesters, National Biology Honor Society; National Psychology Honor Society; Biology Student of the Year (EFGH College); Varsity Lacrosse Player (Michigan State); Outstanding Volunteer Award from St. Mercy Hospital (continued)

10. Extracurricular, Community, and Avocational Activities:

Community activities: Sickle Cell Anemia screening, XY State Univ.

11. Chronological Post-Secondary History, Including Volunteer, Part-Time and Full-time Employment:

Summer 1990 - Lab Technician, Allstate Labs.

1990-91 - Junior Year - Waiter/Cook, Pizza Restaurant - 20 hrs/wk

1996-97 Academic Year - Lab Assistant, Hematology - 15 hrs/wk

Review AMCAS Instructions before completing this form.

29

PERSONAL COMMENTS	Name (Last Name, First Name, MI)
(Your comments must not exceed the space provided. Use a font at least 10 points in size.)	ZYLER, Richard Ross III

#9 cont'd: EFGH College Representative to the National Council on Education in the Sciences

30

SSN 028-26-2288				ACADEMIC RECORD					AMCAS USE ONLY	

Last Name ZYLER				First Name Richard		Middle Name Ross			Suffix III	

College Name Location	Academic Status	BCPM/A	Academic Year	Term	Course Name	Number	Type	Official Transcript Grade	Semester Hours Attempted	AMCAS Grade	AMCAS USE
Bennett College,	FR	A	88	SS	Credit (French)		PF	S	6	P	
Transfer Credit		A			Adv. French Convers			B+			
(Sorbonne/Paris)		A			French Civiliz.(Art)			A			
Bennett College		A		S1	Elementary French		AP		6	G	
Millbrook, N.Y.		A			Intermed French I		AP	B	3	B	
		A			American History		CL		6	L	
		C			Gen Chemistry I+Lab	115		A-	4	A-	
		A			Volleyball	118		A+	1	A	
		A			Philosophy	101		A+	3	A	
		A			Fresh. English Comp	180	H	A-	3	A-	
		P			General Physics I	125		B	4	B	
		M		SM	Calculus I	125		B-	4	B-	
		A		S2	English Literature	109		A	3	A	
		C			Gen Chemistry II+Lab	116		B	4	B	
		A			First Aid & Safety	116		B	2	B	
		A			European History	104		B	3	B	
		M			Calculus II	126		B	4	B	
	SO	P	89	SS	Electromagnetism	103		B	4.5	B	
		A			Literature	131		A-	3	A-	
Nassau Cmty. Col		A		S1	French Literature	001	EX				
Garden City, NY		B			General Biology	201		B+	4	AB	
		C			Organic Chemistry	223		B	3	B	
		A			Medical Ethics	225	AU	NG			
		C			Organic Chem Lab	223		C	1	C	
		B		S2	General Biology	202		B	4	B	
		C			Organic Chemistry	224	PF	S	3	P	
		C			Organic Chem Lab	224	PF	U	1	N	
		A			Social Psychology	227		A	3	A	
		P			General Physics II	222		C+	3	BC	
Michigan State U.	JR	A	90	Q1	Political Science	241		3.5	2.7	AB	
E. Lansing, MI		A			Revolution and War	243	H/I	2.0	2.7	C	
[Narrative		C			Basic Biochemistry	401		3.5	3.3	AB	
Evaluations		B			Comp Vertebrate Anat	314	R	1.0	3.3	D	
Enclosed]		A			Military Drill	259		4.0	0.7	A	
		B		Q2	Comp Vertebrate Anat	314	R	4.0	3.3	A	
		A			Mythology	250		2.0	2.7	C	
		M			Statistics I	201		2.5	2.7	BC	
		A			Modern Ideologies	242		1.5	2.7	CD	
		A		Q3	Anthropology	171		2.0	2.7	C	
		B			Zoology	331		3.0	2.0	B	
		A			Humanities	251		0.0	2.7	F	
Michigan State U.		M	91	QS	Linear Functions	302		3.0	2.7	B	
Study Abroad Prog		A			History of England I	307		4.0	2.7	A	
(Oxfrd/Londn,Eng)		A			Hist of England II	308		2.0	2.7	C	
EFGH College,	SR	M		Q1	Statistics II	91		P	3	C	
Washington, DC		B			Cell & Molec Biol	122		HP	3	B	
		B			Physiology	163		HH	4	A	
		M			Scientific Analysis	22		HH	4	A	
		A			Economics (micro)	2		P	4	C	

Be sure to complete and sign page 4. > >

Achieving the Doctor Dream

College Name Location	Academic Status	BCPM/A	Academic Year	Term	Course Name	Number	Type	Official Transcript Grade	Semester Hours Attempted	AMCAS Grade	AMCAS USE
EFGH College,	SR	B	91	Q2	Med Tech Internship:		PF	CR	16	P	
Washington, DC		B			Hematology	101		86			
Transfer Credit		B			Serology	107		91			
(St. Mercy Hsp,PA)		B			Lab Techniques	111		96			
		B			Virology	113		92			
XY State Univ.	PB	A	92	T1	Occult Literature	120	W	WF			
Washington, DC		A			Tolstoy	220		A	3	A	
		A			Modern Novel	224		A	3	A	
		A	93	T1	Physio. Psychology	301		A	3	A	
		A			Psych. of Learning	304	W	WN			
		A		T2	Research Psychology	340		A	2	A	
		A		T3	Semantics	307	NR	NG	3		
	GR	A	94	T1	Child Psychology	435		A	4	A	
		A			Educ. Psychology	441		B	4	B	
		A		T2	Social Psychology	415		A	4	A	
		A			Abnormal Psychology	460		A	4	A	
		A			Psych. Field Work	490	I	INC	4		
		A	95	T1	Advanced Research	477	PF	PS	4	P	
		A		T2	Death and Dying	503	DG	DF	4		
		A			Advanced Research	477	PF	PS	4	P	
		A		T3	Death and Dying	503		A	4	A	
Abcd University,	GR	M	96	S1	Quantitative Data	668		H	3	A	
Washington, DC		B			Epidemiology	635		HP	4	A-	
		B		S2	Microbiology	665		P	3	B	
		B	97	S1	Biology of Tumors	230	CC		2		
		B			Microbiology	665	CC		3		
		B		S2	Virus Infections	668	CC		1		

---

14. MCAT Testing Status

Number of MCATs taken since April 1991   [3]

Have you taken, or do you plan to take, the August 1997 MCAT?

YES [X]   NO [ ]

15. Medical School

You must answer this Question

[Refer to AMCAS Instructions before answering.] Have you ever matriculated at or attended any medical school as a candidate for the M.D. degree?

YES [ ]   NO [X]

16. Institutional Action

You must answer this Question

[Refer to AMCAS Instructions before answering.] Were you ever the recipient of any action (e.g., dismissal, disqualification, suspension, etc.) by any college or medical school for: (1) unacceptable academic performance or (2) conduct violations? If "YES," explain fully in the "Personal Comments" section (page 2).

YES [ ]   NO [X]

CERTIFICATION STATEMENT

I have read and understand the AMCAS Instructions. I certify that the information submitted in this application and associated materials is current, complete, and accurate to the best of my knowledge.

SIGNATURE (Black Ink Only) or CERTIFICATION

Richard R Tyler III

DATE

June 15, 1997

No. E-6 Rev. 1/97   DCIC No. 97-005   32   COPYRIGHT 1997 BY THE ASSOCIATION OF AMERICAN MEDICAL COLLEGES

AMERICAN MEDICAL COLLEGE APPLICATION SERVICE

ASSOCIATION OF AMERICAN MEDICAL COLLEGES

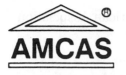

Section for Student Services
2501 M Street, N.W., Lbby-26
Washington, D.C. 20037-1300
Telephone (202) 828-0600

TRANSMITTAL NOTIFICATION (TN)

Your AMCAS Application has been forwarded to the schools listed below, with the biographic and academic information and MCAT scores which appear on this Transmittal Notification (TN). Please check all items carefully and notify AMCAS in writing immediately of any discrepancies. In all correspondence with AMCAS or medical schools, be sure to indicate your complete name, cycle/file number, Social Security Number and telephone number.

```
        10/23/97    Cycle: 090-NEW


To:     RICHARD R ZYLER III                   Soc Sec  #:028-26-2288
        4601 NORTH PARK DR                     Cycle/File #:090-00144
        DAVIS           CA 95616               Entering Class: 1998



        Phone:  916-466-5125                Self Desc: BLACK
        Leg Res:                            Minority/Consider-Ethnic:  YES
             YOLO             CA                        Financial:      NO
        Citizenship: UNITED STATES          Fee Waiver:                NO
        Visa Type:                          Military Service:          NO
        Birth Place: CHEVY CHASE            Previous Med School:       NO
             MONTGOMERY      MD             Institution Action:        NO
        Birthdate: 12/08/70 Age: 26  Sex: MALE
        Num of Dep:                         Early Decision:            NO
                                            Advisor Information Release:YES
Colleges Attended
First 3 Coll on OTI          Major        Program Degree  Degree Dates  Attended
--------- ----------         -----        ------- ------  ------ -----  --------

EFGH COLLEGE                 BIOLOGY      UNDERGR  BS      06/92         89-92

XY ST U MAIN CAMPUS          PSYCHOLOGY   GRADUAT  MA      08/96         92-96

ABCD UNIVERSITY              MICROBIOLOGY GRADUAT  ND                    96-97


          BCPM         AO        Total    MCAT Scores
      GPA   Hours  GPA  Hours GPA  Hours  Test Date(s)      04/97   08/96
FR    3.08  20.0   3.51 18.0 3.28 38.0    Series Number     11      *10
SO    2.97  19.5   3.85  6.0 3.18 25.5
JR    2.83  17.3   2.18 22.3 2.46 39.6    Verbal Reasoning  13-15   12
SR    3.36  14.0   2.00  4.0 3.06 18.0    Physical Sciences 8       7
PBU                4.00 11.0 4.00 11.0    Writing Sample    R       Q
CUG   3.04  70.8   3.05 61.3 3.05 132.1   Biological Sciences 11    10
GRD   3.58  10.0   3.80 20.0 3.73 30.0
                                          *Scores obtained under
                                           nonstandard conditions

    Supplementary Hours:
    Pass/Fail-Pass      33.0              Number of MCAT(S) Taken: 2
    Pass/Fail-Fail       1.0              Next MCAT Date:  08/97
    Advanced Placement   6.0
    CLEP                 6.0

Your Application was    Date of    Yr(s) Prev
Transmitted to:         Application  Applied

Code    School
 849 XYZ MED SCHOOL     101897           97
 850 ABC MED SCHOOL     101897         96,95
#851 DEF MED COLLEGE    101897     97,96,95,94@
 855 MTM MED COLLEGE    101897
 857 JKL MED SCHOOL     101897         97,94@

# State law prohibits distribution of information on sex, date of birth, and age
  to this medical school for admissions consideration.
@ Represents application to and/or application prior to this entering class year.
```

Reference Section

AACOMAS *Instruction Booklet: 1998 Entering Class.* Chevy Chase, MD: American Association of Colleges of Osteopathic Medicine, 1997.

AMCAS *Instruction Booklet for the 1998 Entering Class.* Washington, DC: Association of American Medical Colleges, 1997.

13

Letters of Recommendation
Your Personal Essay

Recommendations

One of the most important aspects of your application will be the letters of recommendation provided by both your professors and premedical advisor. If a premedical advisory committee is evaluating your file, there will still usually be one person responsible for writing your final letter. In some cases, it may also be appropriate to have others write letters (*e.g.* an employer or person who knows you well from other activities such as volunteer work, research, extracurricular activities, etc.) on your behalf. Medical schools are usually specific about their requests regarding letters of recommendation and will inform you about what types of letters should be sent. Besides the premedical advisory letter, medical schools usually ask for an additional two or three letters of recommendation. If a medical school allows additional letters to be sent, the admissions office will usually be specific about limiting the number of these letters.

The premedical advisory letter will be written about the "whole" person—not just about your academic accomplishments, but also your personal attributes and qualities that will make you an asset to the medical profession. The premed advisor/committee will usually have your complete file (grade transcripts, MCAT scores, letters of recommendation, a current resumé, your personal essay) so that a thorough letter can be written on your behalf (As a general rule, letters of recommendation are usually one to two pages long.). This letter from the premed advisory office may also contain one or more brief statements from your other recommendation letters in your academic file. If, for example, your chemistry or physics professor wrote about your stellar performance in a course, the comments would probably be highlighted in the premedical advisory letter. A discussion of honors, awards, and extracurricular activities would also be included and would portray the applicant's unique qualities and contributions. An evaluation of any problem or inconsistencies in an applicant's record could also be discussed in such a letter.

It is important to obtain letters of recommendation from professors who know you as a person and not just as one of the students who received an "A" in a certain class. If the professor knows your personal characteristics and attributes, a more effective letter can be written because it will provide insight about you as a person and a "future doctor." The comment that a student received "one of the highest grades" is very helpful, but knowing that he/she was one of the most dedicated and motivated students in class can be more insightful.

When you request letters of recommendation to be written, ask the professors if they will write favorable ones on your behalf. This may seem obvious to the applicant, but it is an extremely important factor that could directly affect your application. A negative letter could hurt the student's chances for both interviews and admission into medical school. If a professor feels that he/she cannot write a positive letter or feels "uncomfortable" writing about someone he/she "does not really know," then do not request a letter from that person.

The timing of your requests is also crucial. It will be important for your file to be complete early so that delays in the application process can be avoided. The ideal time to have those letters written is during the spring or summer of your application year. Your requests for the letters should therefore occur before the end of your academic year. It is extremely important to personalize this effort—set up an appointment to see the professor. . . . Be organized, on-time, and dress appropriately! Make sure you schedule enough time for this appointment so that you can discuss your career plans. If the professor does agree to write you a letter, you can then provide a copy of a current resumé and a list of names/addresses to where these letters should be sent. Some undergraduate schools have a "centralized processing system"—all the letters of recommendation are mailed together to each individual school designated by the applicant. At this initial meeting with your recommenders, you will probably not have a complete list of addresses (Medical schools using AMCAS will send you further information regarding letters of recommendation once your application is processed.). It will be important to update these addresses and to provide the information to both the premedical advisory office and those writing your letters of recommendation. These letters can be written earlier in the application process and then can be sent as the address/contact information is updated. As an applicant, you should also send thank-you letters to your instructors and others who write letters of recommendation on your behalf. You should also keep them updated on your progress during the application year and personally inform them once you are accepted into medical school.

The Personal Essay

Another key factor in obtaining both an interview and an acceptance letter will be your personal essay. The AMCAS form and many non-AMCAS schools usually allow approximately one full page for the applicant to submit a typewritten personal essay. There are a number of helpful hints that can guide you in writing both an effective and well-written personal statement:

1. Before even attempting the first words of the essay, you should write down your ideas and themes in outline form. You need to think carefully about the different approaches you may

take in writing the essay. It is important to keep an open mind about the variety of themes that are possible for an essay of this type. (Remember, there are many approaches to writing a successful essay.) You may even find yourself writing a few outlines and essays before deciding on the one that will convey your message to the reader.

2. Writing about your decision to become a doctor and the qualities that are necessary to be a physician are examples of two themes that are commonly discussed in the personal statement. Incorporating your life experiences and personal qualities and attributes into this general framework can make the essay both interesting and unique. Your personal statement, in essence, should have "its own personality"—one which can set you apart from other candidates seeking admission into medical school.

3. Your experiences can relate to such factors as family life, extracurricular activities, employment, and volunteer activities (to name a few)—all of which have helped mold you into that unique person that you are!

4. There are your own personal qualities and attributes that you may want to highlight for the reader. Leadership abilities, working well with others, exhibiting motivation, perseverance, and/or discipline, being a compassionate person—these are only a few illustrations of one or more personal qualities that you may choose to discuss about yourself in the essay.

5. Do not use the essay to write down "the obvious." If you have listed honors, awards, and activities elsewhere in the application, do not waste valuable essay space by repeating what the reader already knows about you. It would, of course, be appropriate and essential to discuss one of your previously listed achievements if your intention is to discuss an important life experience or personal quality.

6. As with any well-written statement or story, the first few sentences usually determine whether or not you can obtain and keep the reader's attention. Though every sentence is important in this type of essay, it will be important to have strong first and last paragraphs so that the reader can maintain a good overall impression of the applicant.

7. Your written communication skills and abilities will also be exhibited through your personal statement. Make sure the grammatical usage, spelling, syntax, and punctuation are correct. . . . You need to pay attention to these details because problems in these areas of writing could cost you a potential interview. It may be necessary to work through different

revisions and draft copies of your statement, but the time and effort will be worth it in the end!

8. Accentuate the positive. . . . If you need to explain a potential problem, discrepancy, or weakness in your application—concentrate on the favorable aspects and factors. If you, for example, received a "C" in general physics, you can prove your perseverance and motivation by showing that you made a great "come-back" on the MCAT by scoring an "11" on the Physical Sciences Section.

If you were rejected from medical school the first time around, concentrate on the experiences in your life which have since further strengthened your desire to become a doctor—volunteer work with patients, obtaining excellent grades in extra coursework such as physiology or biochemistry (or other medical related basic science coursework). . . . The year(s) between college and medical school can be shown as a time of personal growth and development. . . . You should write about your experiences honestly and in a positive manner.

9. Those who have had other careers before deciding on medicine should also concentrate on the positive aspects and experiences of what they have already learned. There are numerous skills (e.g. leadership ability; working with people; counseling others; good writing abilities, etc.) that can also be applicable and very helpful in the practice of medicine.

10. Do not be egotistical or boastful. . . . "Pompous" language which enhances your accomplishments could turn off both the reader and a future opportunity for an interview. It is important to be proud of your accomplishments (Do not minimize them!) but discussing them with a more "toned down approach" should impress the reader in a more favorable and positive manner.

11. Getting other people to read your essay is also a good idea. Your essay's theme(s)/message(s) should be clearly communicated to the reader. Do not hesitate to allow others to critique your writing ability—remember that the extra effort you put into your final draft may get you that interview!

12. Secondary applications commonly ask for additional short answers or essays about a variety of topics. You may, for example, be asked to write about one of your extracurricular activities or one of your employment experiences. Remember to answer the specific question that is being asked.

13. Remember to follow directions closely and write your personal statement or additional essays (for secondary applications) in the allotted space. Do not send additional sheets with your secondary application unless the medical school allows extra space for your answers/ essays.

14. Before you actually submit your final copy, make sure there are no "typos" in the personal essay.

15. Remember to read, study, and re-read your essay before you go for your interview(s). It is very likely that you will be asked one or more specific questions about the content of your essay.

14

Interviewing: "The Time To Shine"

The medical school interview will be the most important interview in the initiation of your professional career. A composite objective picture of your record has already been carefully looked at—GPAs, MCAT scores, letters of recommendation, essays—these factors have given the committee a glimpse of your accomplishments. The interview, however, will look at WHO AND WHAT YOU REALLY ARE ABOUT! Being asked to interview has automatically put you in that school's group of students who are considered "most competitive" for admission. Of course, this group will even have its own "subsets" of students. There will be those with "cream of the crop credentials" (academic, research, and personality "stars")—those who will get admitted to every school they apply and interview at; unless a student in this category interviews poorly, a medical school will look at the interview as an "active recruitment session" in order to portray the school's strength. There is also the large group of students who have excellent grades and MCATs. Do you wonder how medical schools can choose among all those applicants with 3.5–3.6 GPAs and 10s on their MCAT? . . . The INTERVIEW, of course, will help make the difference. There are also a large number of students with qualifying grades and scores who have other strong credentials or unique factors in their background. Again, the interview will be a very important factor in gaining admission.

Medical school admission committees want to attract "quality people" for their entering class. The interview, in this sense, also serves as an opportunity for both the medical school and the applicant to get to know each other. The interviewing process literally works both ways (It is NOT A ONE-WAY STREET!). . . . There is a "give and take". . . . A chance for the applicant to "interview" the medical school in order to find out all relevant information so that he/she can make a decision about where to spend the next very important four years.

In summary, the interviewing process has two major goals:

1. Getting to know the "whole person." The "personal side" of the candidate can tell more than just what appears on paper.

2. Recruitment of the entering class involves "marketing the medical school." This is accomplished in a number of ways on "interview days": Tours of the facilities, library, labs, informal

---

question and answer sessions, discussions with medical students, questioning the interviewer(s) about the school, etc.

There is a long list of factors that any medical school interviewer may try to evaluate in the applicant/interviewee. Though every area cannot be considered in a thirty minute interview, you would be surprised by how many of them actually do get evaluated. The following list attempts to give the interviewee an excellent idea of what is evaluated.

Characteristics/Qualities/Additional Criteria That Are Evaluated

1. Your interest and motivation for wanting to become a doctor
2. Communication skills
3. Interpersonal skills
4. Maturity
5. Compassionate/empathetic
6. Motivation/perseverance
7. Leadership abilities
8. Energy level
9. Sense of humor
10. Character
11. Polite/respectful
12. Honesty
13. Appearance
14. Good listener
15. Emotional stability/personal composure
16. Friendly
17. Ability to relate to others
18. General knowledge
19. Being a "positive thinker"
20. Confidence level
21. Personal enthusiasm/enthusiasm about this medical school

22. Outside interests and hobbies

23. Honors and awards

24. Volunteer service (health care or non-health care related)

25. Work experience (paid and volunteer)

26. Research experience (if applicable)

27. Health care related experience

28. Other extracurricular activities

Interviewers may ask more specific questions about the content of your formal application. Some of these areas will have been covered in your written application (*e.g.* work experience, extracurricular activities, honors and awards, etc.). . . . You may be asked, for example, to explain your personal responsibilities, leadership roles, and interests in a certain activity.

Interview Preparation

There is NO SUBSTITUTE FOR PREPARATION. By being well prepared, you will be more confident and relaxed on the actual day of your interview. There are a number of preparation methods that will help you make the most of your interview day(s). Remember that success cannot be absolutely guaranteed, but it can be well NURTURED!

1. RE-READ AND KNOW EVERYTHING IN YOUR APPLICATION MATERIALS.

    You don't want to act surprised or look like you are "fumbling for an answer" when a specific question is asked about the content of your formal application. EVERYTHING should be examined carefully: AMCAS application, personal essay, secondary application (including all additional essays and short answer responses), and non-AMCAS application (for those specific schools).

2. READ AND STUDY ALL MATERIALS (CATALOGS, BROCHURES, PAMPHLETS) SENT BY THE INTERVIEWING SCHOOLS.

    It will give you a knowledge base to ask appropriate and informational questions about the medical school. What's more, your familiarity with that medical school can give a very favorable impression in the eyes of the interviewer. Remember that medical school interviewers want to fill their entering class with students who are "suitable for their school." (Many interviewers ask: "Why this medical school?" "What interests you in this medical school?")

3. INVOLVE YOURSELF IN A MOCK INTERVIEW.

Premedical advisors, professors, and other premedical students can give you a trial "run-through" in preparation for the "real thing." Make a list of common (and "not so common") questions that might be asked at your medical school interview. The next chapter has numerous sample questions that can serve as a detailed guideline for your preparation.

Many college premedical advisory departments and college career placement offices offer formal mock interviews. (Some will even provide a videotaped practice interview so that you and your advisors can critique your performance.) If there is not a formal mock interview program at your school, consider asking advisors, instructors, or other premedical students who are also applying to medical school to participate in your own informal program. Friends and relatives may also be excellent sources to help you with these practice sessions.

When you do a mock interview, you should allow the interviewer to be candid about your performance: "first impressions," verbal critiques, and detailed written evaluations by the interviewer(s) will all help you improve your performance for the actual interview.

Practice interviews will allow you to key in on everything from body mannerisms to the substance and accuracy of your answers.

4. MAKE YOUR UNDERGRADUATE PREMED CLUB WORK FOR THE APPLICANTS' ADVANTAGE.

At some colleges, the premedical advisory committee and/or the premed club compile "feedback questionnaires" that are answered voluntarily by the interviewees. Students are encouraged to answer the questionnaire in sufficient detail about each of the medical schools they had interviewed. The forms are usually completed shortly after the interview so the experience is still "fresh in everyone's mind" and specific questions can be remembered. Some questionnaires even ask about the interviewers' names and "interviewing style" so that other applicants can be "well prepared." Knowing the medical school's itinerary (tours, information sessions, length of interviews, etc.) ahead of time also helps to inspire confidence and keep the applicant more relaxed about the interview day.

If this service is not available at your school, take the initiative to compare notes with other premed students who are getting interviews. Chances are that you will be interviewing at some of the same schools—especially the medical schools in your state.

5. MAKE SURE YOU ARE UP TO DATE ON CURRENT EVENTS AND "HEALTH CARE" NEWS.

It is important to periodically watch the national news and to skim a newspaper. The national news magazines are also excellent resources. (They usually have separate sections on health affairs.) You do not have to go overboard by reading everything. . . . The "awareness factor" dictates that you should selectively "pick and choose" articles that cover the "hot topics" of the day (especially those related to health care: managed care, health care legislation, HMOs, medical/legal/ethical issues, etc.).

6. KNOW THE REASONS WHY YOU WANT TO BECOME A PHYSICIAN.

Think carefully about the people, events, or other factors in your life that may have influenced your career decision. Your motivation and reasons for wanting to be a doctor are probably the most common questions asked by interviewers.

7. REVIEW THE DETAILS OF YOUR PERSONAL ESSAY (AND OTHER ESSAYS THAT YOU MAY HAVE WRITTEN ON SECONDARY APPLICATIONS).

This is another very common area that serves as a source for interviewer questions.

8. PREPARE ANSWERS TO SOME OF THE POTENTIAL QUESTIONS YOU MAY BE ASKED.

It is a very good idea to write down/outline your answers to some of the more common questions you might be asked. . . . This allows you to get in the right frame of mind for the interview. Do not just write down and "internalize your prospective answers" . . . VOICE THEM OUT. . . . This will give you additional practice. At the same time, however, you do not want to present yourself at the medical school interview with "memorized answers". . . . With "canned answers," your style may appear "stifled". . . . Interviewers have a keen sense to an interviewee's style, and it is to your advantage to appear "natural and spontaneous."

Knowing the Logistics of Medical School Interviews

1. <u>You will usually have a full day of activities scheduled around your actual interviews.</u>

An orientation session or a short meeting with an admissions office person will provide you with the day's itinerary: times of your interviews (names of the interviewers are usually also provided), information sessions, tours (medical school facilities, library, sometimes hospitals or clinics), lunch, opportunities to meet with medical students, attend a class, etc.

2. Medical schools schedule "interview days."

    There will be a number of other applicants with you on that day. Do not let others affect you by playing into the "intimidation game." There may be informal talk among the interviewees about GPAs/ MCAT scores/ "extraordinary achievements"/where they have been interviewed and have been accepted, etc. . . . Remember to JUST BE YOURSELF . . . . That medical school where you received the interview has room for qualified applicants, and YOU ARE ONE OF THEM!

3. Interviews.

    You will have interviews by one or more members of the following categories:

    - "Basic science" faculty (These are instructors who teach in the first two years of the medical school curriculum.) This will include mostly Ph.D.'s and perhaps some M.D.'s.
    - Clinical faculty: M.D.'s from the various departments: Internal medicine, surgery, pediatrics, obstetrics and gynecology, etc.
    - Members of the administration
    - Researchers (M.D.'s, Ph.D.'s, M.D./Ph.D.'s)
    - M.D. alumni/ae
    - Medical students

4. Duration and number of interviews.

    The "typical" interview lasts thirty to forty-five minutes. Interviews, however, can range from twenty minutes to one hour. The average number of interviews is usually two; you may, however, have anywhere from one to four or more interviews (includes group/panel interviews where a number of people may be asking questions).

5. Interview Types.

    1. OPEN INTERVIEWS

        The interviewer has access to your application file and has reviewed/studied it. The interviewer usually brings the application and may directly refer to it during your meeting. Sometimes the interviewer does not have access to your entire application but has read your personal statement.

    2. CLOSED INTERVIEWS

        Your interviewer will not have access to your application. This interviewer will typically ask open-ended and informational questions to find out more about you.

3. GROUP INTERVIEWS

These types of interviews are the exception and not the rule. A group of interviewers may talk to you alone or with a small group (usually two to three) of applicants. Do not be INTIMIDATED by this type of interview. . . . Look at it as an effective way of presenting both your personal attributes and your ability to interact well with a diverse group of people.

4. REGIONAL INTERVIEWS (WITH ADMISSIONS OFFICERS OR ALUMNI)

These interviews are sometimes offered to students who may be geographically distant from the medical school. It is a means of saving time and money, but the "personal expense" is that you will not be able to talk with faculty and students or see what the school has to really offer (geographical setting, facilities, labs, hospitals, etc.). If you are seriously interested in attending the school and are accepted (after having a "regional interview"), you should make every effort to visit. Remember, this is the start of your medical career, and you need to match a medical school's "overall personality" with your interests.

Be Aware of Interviewer Styles

ONE or MORE of the following styles/methods may be used during your actual interview. No matter which ones are used, the interviewers will be carefully looking at your abilities, personal characteristics, interpersonal skills, and a myriad of factors that were first listed at the beginning of this chapter.

1. "INFORMATIONAL" INTERVIEW

Simply put, the interviewer will ask you to clarify a number of points in your written application that may be ambiguous or have insufficient detail. (There is usually insufficient space on an application, for example, to discuss in detail your extracurricular activities, work history, honors and awards.) Though these questions appear to be "straightforward," remember that a host of other factors such as communication ability and personal qualities are being scrutinized. This style of interview is also very common when you are in a "closed interview"—the interviewer does not have access to your formal application so he/she is inclined to ask "open-ended" informational questions about yourself.

2. ISSUES AND OPINIONS

Some interviewers will ask very little about the content of your application. (They have already seen your GPA, MCAT scores, essays, and other data and choose not to ask about them.) Their main objective may be to see if you communicate well and if you can "think on your feet."

3. ARGUMENTATIVE/"DISAGREEABLE" STYLE

Some interviewers may outwardly disagree with your opinions or viewpoints. DO NOT OVERREACT to this type of interviewing style. . . . DO NOT TAKE IT PERSONALLY! The practice of medicine can be quite stressful at times, and the interviewer wants to test your reaction to such a situation. What's more, interviewers will be more concerned about your critical/logical thought processes than the "right" or the "wrong" opinion or viewpoint.

4. MOST INTERVIEWERS WILL LEAVE TIME TO ANSWER YOUR QUESTIONS ABOUT THE MEDICAL SCHOOL.

You should ask well-informed and "appropriate" questions. (Avoid asking "obvious questions" that can be answered by reading a brochure.) Asking an interviewer about his/her specialty, medical practice, or research is also appropriate (especially if you have a genuine common interest in some of those areas).

"Rules of Advice" for a Good Medical School Interview

1. <u>Eat an energizing breakfast.</u>

Cereal, oatmeal, juice, and fruit are excellent choices. . . . Remember, coffee may exacerbate nervousness or anxiety.

2. <u>Leave negative personal qualities/characteristics behind at the interview door.</u>

If you portray yourself as pretentious/obnoxious/argumentative or even shy/introverted, your chances for admission will be diminished.

3. <u>Be a positive thinker.</u>

Stay confident about your attributes and accomplishments. Making it to an interview is an achievement that puts you one step away from acceptance. Remember, MEDICAL SCHOOLS INTERVIEW PEOPLE THEY ARE INTERESTED IN!

4. <u>Be polite and friendly.</u>

Personal indiscretions such as being discourteous to a secretary, staff member, medical student, or interviewer is inexcusable! ("Treat others like you would want to be treated.") Any "behavioral miscues" have a way of making their way back to an admissions committee and would definitely hurt your chance of admission.

5. <u>Be a good listener; address the questions being asked.</u>

If you think that you don't understand the question or don't know an answer. . . . Don't be afraid to say so! It is much better to be honest and truthful than to ramble relentlessly or fumble with an insincere answer.

6. <u>If you have a genuine interest in attending that medical school, SHOW IT!</u>

BE ENTHUSIASTIC (but "not artificially so"); ask appropriate questions and exhibit some detailed knowledge about the school. Remember, medical schools have "personalities of their own" and want to fill their first-year class with students SUITABLE FOR THEIR SCHOOL!

7. <u>Timeliness is of utmost importance.</u>

You will have a long, busy day filled with different activities. If you have to break away from lunch or an information session, politely excuse yourself and go for your scheduled interview.

To save yourself time and to avoid anxiety, make sure you know where the actual interview rooms are. You will have some free time during the day, so take the initiative and find where your interviews will be. There is nothing worse than being late, anxious, and disheveled because you spent five to ten minutes of your allotted interviewing time looking for the room.

8. <u>Be truthful, straightforward, and ethical; do not exaggerate!</u>

Human nature may whisper in your ear to put yourself in the BEST ABSOLUTE POSSIBLE LIGHT. . . . This is NOT ACCOMPLISHED by BEING EVASIVE but by BEING HONEST! Your interviewer, for example, may specifically address a weakness in your academic record (a low grade or course withdrawals). Approach the question directly and "tell it as it is." Interviewers have a keen sense of when an applicant may be attempting to avoid an answer; "EVASIVENESS" could very well get you a rejection letter.

9. <u>Make effective use of any free time during the interview schedule.</u>

Attending a class, talking with medical students about the school and its location, looking at school billboards to learn about student activities—those will all give you extra insight into the "personality of that school."

Attempt to get all of your questions answered. Consider what the community has to offer and also look at the cost of living issues. Medical students are an excellent source of information on such issues as rental costs and about what to do in the geographical area with available free time.

10. <u>Look professional, dress professional.</u>

Be well groomed and dress conservatively. Avoid too bright and flowery colors and patterns. Make sure your shoes are shined! Women should avoid excessive makeup and excessive amounts of jewelry ("EXCESSIVE" translates into a DISTRACTION!).

11. <u>Greet your interviewer with a SMILE, a FIRM HANDSHAKE, and GOOD EYE CONTACT.</u>

12. <u>Maintain good eye contact during the interview.</u>

13. <u>Maintain good posture (No slouching!) and avoid nervous habits and mannerisms.</u>

14. <u>If you need to stay overnight</u>. . . . Inquire about any available discount rates (on campus or at hotels). Sometimes arrangements can be made to stay with a medical student. This can serve as an excellent opportunity to learn what medical school is really all about.

15. <u>Obtain directions to the school.</u>

If you need a campus map, ask or write for one.

16. <u>Direct questions to your interviewer about the medical school.</u>

17. <u>Direct questions to your interviewer about his/her specialty or research (especially if you have a common interest). Also ask the interviewer how he/she likes living in this geographic location.</u>

Questions such as those help contribute to the "personal flavor" of a formal interview and can sometimes even help form a "common bond" between the interviewer and the applicant.

18. <u>Avoid getting angry or showing frustration with your interviewer</u>.

Some interviewers may disagree or question some or all of your viewpoints or answers. Remember, they want to see your reaction under a stressful situation. (You may feel "insulted or betrayed," but DO NOT ACT LIKE IT IS an unfair situation.) SHOW YOUR MATURITY AND LEVEL-HEADEDNESS!

19. <u>Know the pronunciation of your interviewers' names</u>.

You will usually receive an itinerary at the beginning of the day that will list the interviewers' names. (If they are not given, politely ask an appropriate person about the interviewers' names.) If you are unsure about a pronunciation, ask an admission's office secretary or any of the people who are in charge of the various activities for the day. Also, listen carefully to when the interviewer introduces himself/herself. (That, of course, will be the exact pronunciation.)

20. <u>Mail a typed "thank you" letter to each of your interviewers</u>.

Highlight specific areas or issues that were covered in each interview. Remember to thank them for the school's hospitality (tours, lunch, informational sessions, etc.). You should also write about some of the school's attributes and address the major reasons for wanting to attend that medical school.

A general "etiquette rule for medical school interviewing" is that you should wait for the school's formal interview invitation. An exception to this rule is requesting an interview from a particular school when you have another interview(s) in the same geographical area. This may save you a considerable amount of time and money during your interviewing schedule. If you do request an interview under those circumstances, it is MANDATORY that you again SHOW THE PROPER ETIQUETTE. Make your formal request in writing to the Admissions Committee (either the Director of Admissions or the Dean of Admissions) informing them that you have interviews—name the school(s) and the date(s)—in the geographical area. If "time is short," you can telephone the school but immediately follow that up with a letter. Ask them to review your file for a possible interview. Be "upbeat and enthusiastic" but never act "pushy" or demanding. That medical school will usually review your file and give you a reply before your interview trip to that geographical area.

15

Food For Thought: Questions to Consider For Your Medical School Interview

Personal Matters

1. Please tell me about yourself. (Tell me about [your name].)

2. Tell me about your family.

3. Tell me about your parents.

4. Tell me about your sisters/brothers.

5. Are there physicians in your family? Have they influenced your decision to become a doctor?

6. Please discuss your grade school years.

7. Talk to me about your high school years.

8. What are your personal strengths?

9. What are your personal weaknesses?

10. What are your outside interests/hobbies?

11. Where did you spend your early years?

12. Do you have a favorite book? (Why that book?)

13. What do you do with your free time?

14. What do you do when you get upset/angry?

15. What has been the biggest event in your life so far? Why?

16. Do you have a favorite sport?

17. What do you see yourself doing 10 (or 20) years from now?

18. Would you change anything in your life? What would you do differently?

19. Tell me about a proud accomplishment.

20. How would your best friend describe you?

21. Specific questions about your personal essay.

22. Specific questions about personal answers from the secondary application.

23. Who has been the most influential person in your life?

24. What do you do for exercise?

25. Is there anything else I should know about you?

26. Do you plan on having a family? How will you mix a family life with a career?

27. Do you have a spouse/children? How do they feel about your plans to attend medical school?

28. Did you ever have a terminally ill relative or friend?

29. What have been the biggest changes in your life since you attended high school?

30. What single personal characteristic got you to this point in your life?

Interest in Medicine/Motivation for Becoming a Physician

1. Why do you want to be a doctor?

2. Did any event(s) in your life influence you to become a doctor?

3. What area/specialty of medicine would you like to go into?

4. What qualities do you look for in a good physician?

5. What would be your second career choice if you did not want to be a doctor? Why?

6. Tell me about your activities that have exposed you to medicine.

7. Have you worked in a hospital/clinic?

8. When did you decide to become a physician?

9. Did your parents play a role in your decision to become a doctor?

10. What are your parents' thoughts about your interests in medical school?

11. Do you want to work in a solo practice/small group/large group/hospital practice/HMO practice?

12. When you start to practice medicine, what type of geographic area (large city/suburban/ medium-small town/rural) would you like to live in? Why?

13. Do you personally know any physicians? Have they influenced your decision to attend medical school?

14. Why is the practice of medicine both "an art and a science"?

15. When you become a doctor, how will you handle a patient who is not compliant?

16. How do you think a doctor spends his/her average day?

17. Why medicine. . . and not dentistry, podiatry, or public health?

18. Are you mainly interested in a clinical or research career?

College Years

1. Why did you attend your college?

2. Discuss your extracurricular activities.

3. What is your favorite extracurricular activity? Why?

4. Why did you major in _____?

5. Tell me about your favorite course.

6. What was your least favorite course in college? Why?

7. What leadership roles have you held?

8. Tell me about your research/research project (if applicable).

9. Why did your GPA fall during the _____ semester?

10. How have you spent your summers?

11. Tell me about this particular job.

12. How did you finance your undergraduate education?

13. What happened that your MCAT scores increased/decreased the second time?

14. What did you do to prepare for the MCAT?

15. What happened that you got a "C" in organic chemistry?

16. What makes an effective teacher?

17. If you hadn't majored in _____, what would have been your second choice? Why?

18. If you had to do it all over again, would you attend the same college or go elsewhere?

Personal Qualities/Characteristics

1. What are the qualities of a mature individual?

2. What makes a person a quality leader?

3. How do you deal with failure?

4. How do you handle difficult times in your life?

5. How do you handle emotionally sad times in your life?

6. How do you handle embarrassment? (Can you give me an example from your life?)

7. How do you deal with argumentative/disagreeable people?

8. How do you handle criticism?

9. What do you like most about your best friend?

10. What has been your biggest challenge? How did you respond?

11. What qualities would you like to see in a co-worker?

12. How do you cope with stress?

13. How do you handle upset/angry people?

14. Could you give me two words that might describe yourself?

15. What does it mean to be a team player? What personal qualities make a person a team player?

Medical School Application Issues

1. Why do you want to attend this medical school?

2. Why should this medical school accept you?

3. Do you know how tough medical school is? Are you prepared for the demands of medical school?

4. What medical schools have you applied to? Where have you been interviewed?

5. If medical schools reject you this year, what will you do?

6. How will you finance your medical school education?

7. How do you think your life will change when you start medical school?

8. What should I tell the admissions committee about you?

9. If you are accepted by more than one medical school, how will you decide on which one to attend?

Viewpoints on Health Care Issues/Health Affairs

1. What is an HMO? What do you know about HMOs and their effect(s) on the practice of medicine?

2. What is a PPO?

3. How do you define "managed care"?

4. What is your view on national health insurance?

5. Do you have any views on national health care reform?

6. Is the practice of medicine becoming too "business-like"?

7. Is government trying to involve itself too much in our health care system?

8. Are physicians' incomes excessive?

9. Are you aware of any recent legislation regarding health care reform?

10. Do you think there is a medical malpractice crisis?

11. What if you got sued?

12. Do you think our legal system is an effective one?

13. Could you give me an example(s) of one or more countries which have "socialized medicine"? Would their system(s) work in the United States?

14. Is there really a "physician surplus"? If there is one, what should we do about it?

15. What is meant by primary care? Do you know what one or more of the primary care specialties are?

16. What is our country's biggest problem today? What should we do about it?

Medical Ethics/Medical-Legal Matters

1. Does a person have a right to free health care?

2. Do you have an opinion about abortion?

3. What do you think about physician-assisted suicide?

4. Do you have a viewpoint on animal experimentation/research?

5. How do you feel about treating poor patients/uninsured patients?

6. How do you feel about treating an AIDS patient?

7. What is a living will?

8. What is a "durable power of attorney with a health care proxy "?

Current Events/Current Issues

1. What is your opinion on _____ (a current event)?

2. Should the U.S. have a constitutional amendment to balance the budget? Why/Why not?

3. How should we balance the budget? What should our national priorities be in balancing the budget?

4. Should there be term limits for congressmen/women? Why/Why not?

5. What is your view on the tobacco industry?

Other Assorted Questions

1. Do you have any questions for me today?

2. Is there anything you would like to know about me?

3. If you suddenly won the lottery, what would you do?

4. What types of movies do you like?

5. What type of music do you like?

16

Questions You Should Ask About Medical Schools

The opportunity to learn all you can about a medical school is important for both your interview and your decision on where to attend. Initially, it will also be extremely beneficial in helping you decide where to apply to medical school. Interview day will give you an opportunity to speak with students and faculty and also to take tours of buildings, labs, libraries, and perhaps even one of the clinical sites. Knowing all you can about a medical school will allow you to get a better "feel" for the school's "personality" once you actually visit. Your knowledge about the school and your impressions from interview day will also be major factors in helping you decide WHICH MEDICAL SCHOOL IS RIGHT FOR YOU!

During your application year, you will be inundated with a variety of resources about medical school—brochures, pamphlets, catalogs, bulletins, and flyers—all of this information should be carefully read and reviewed. There is a large amount of facts that you can learn from all of these informational sources. These categories of information are numerous and include the following (You can also use this listing as your own checklist when organizing all of the medical school information):

1. History of the medical school and the affiliated university (if the medical school is part of an extended university system).

2. Description of the geographical area and the available opportunities (recreational, cultural, cost of living, etc.).

3. Course requirements for admission.

4. Admission selection factors.

5. GPAs/MCAT scores.

6. Class size.

7. Class demographics:
    - Average age/age range
    - Percentage of men/women
    - Percentage minority (African-American/American-Indian/Mexican-American/Mainland Puerto Rican)
    - Percentage of state residents/non-state residents
    - Types of college majors
    - Class degrees (B.A., B.S., M.S., Ph.D.s, etc.)

8. Application dates and deadlines:
    - Application filing (earliest/latest dates)
    - AMCAS or non-AMCAS school
    - Application fee
    - Secondary application information
        1. Letters of recommendation
        2. Additional information
        3. Additional essays/short answers
    - Acceptance notices to applicants (earliest/latest dates)
    - Maximum time response to accept an offer of admission
    - Deposit (money) requirements to hold a class position
    - Starting date for the first-year class
    - Availability of an Early Decision Plan

9. Number of applicants/number or percentage of applicants interviewed

10. Description of the curriculum
    a) Basic science course list
    b) Clinical clerkships

11. Estimated annual cost of medical school (tuition/fees/cost of living expenses, etc.)

12. Financial aid (scholarships/grants/loans)

13. Armed Forces' scholarships

14. Government sponsored scholarship programs

15. B.S/M.D. programs

16. Joint Degree Programs

17. Research opportunities for students

18. Availability of special pathways (three-year or five-year M.D. programs)

19. Information on interviews

20. Information on transfer and/or advanced standing students

21. Specific information on hospitals

23. Availability of summer programs

24. Grading/evaluation policies

25. Immunization requirements for students

During your interview day, you will have a unique opportunity for finding answers to your specific medical school questions. Your faculty interviewers, along with medical students who are made available to answer questions, will be your main sources. There may also be formal question and answer seminars available for the interviewees (or an "informal" session during lunch).

There are some questions that will not be answered just by looking at written information. There are also other questions that you will seek further information or explanation based on what you have already read or heard about that particular medical school. You also need to ask the appropriate questions to the "proper" person. You should not ask the faculty interviewer about the "average student rent" or about the "typical" social activities of medical students. Questions, for example, about the academic curriculum or passage rates on national board examinations would be more appropriate.

The following list serves as sample questions you should consider when evaluating a medical school. It is a "thorough list" but still only serves to provide GOOD FOOD FOR YOUR OWN THOUGHTS AND QUESTIONS.

Sample Questions to Ask or Consider
When Evaluating a Medical School

1. Is your medical school nationally known for any of its medical specialties or research?

2. What are the medical school's strongest basic medical science departments? What are the weakest departments? Why?

3. What are the strongest clinical medical departments?

4. What is the passing rate for the second-year class on the first part of the national medical boards (a/k/a the USMLE Step 1 [the United States Medical Licensing Examination])? Is passing USMLE Step 1 a prerequisite before going on to your third year of medical school? Is passing USMLE Step 2 a prerequisite to receiving an M.D. degree from that medical school?

5. If a student does not pass either USMLE Step 1 or USMLE Step 2, what type of scheduling arrangements are made?

6. Is tutoring available for those who do not pass their national board exams the first time around?

7. Is tutoring available for students having difficulty with courses during the regular academic year?

8. If a student does not pass a course, what arrangements are made to repeat the course—in the summer or next academic year?

9. Does the school provide any auxiliary services to help students prepare for the national board examinations (USMLE Step 1 and Step 2)?

10. How many students drop out, transfer, or take leaves of absence per year? What are the main reasons?

11. How many students leave that medical school based on their academic performance?

12. Is there a faculty/student advisory system at your school? Do you have the same advisor all four years? Is there a separate basic sciences curriculum advisor and a clinical clerkship advisor?

13. Do second-year students serve as advisors to first-year students?

14. Are any electives available during the first two years of the basic medical science curriculum?

15. Are there courses that will expose me to medical ethics, medical-legal issues, and the business side of medicine?

16. What are the required clinical clerkships during the fourth year of medical school?

17. Can fourth year clinical clerkship electives be taken at other hospitals (e.g. in another city or state)? What is the maximum number of such electives?

18. How early in my medical school career do I get formally exposed to clinical medicine?

19. How are students evaluated during their clinical years?

20. What is the "residency match" all about?

21. What percentage of fourth-year medical students get their top residency (specialty/hospital) choice?. . . their second choice (hospital)?. . . or their third choice (hospital)?

22. Is it possible to see a residency appointment list (by specialty/hospital) for recent graduates of your medical school?

23. What types of arrangements are made for those who do not initially "match" for a residency position?

24. How much time is allowed during the fourth year to interview for a residency position?

25. Does your school emphasize the primary care specialties?

26. Could you tell me about the school's basic science curriculum? Is it "traditional"/based on the "systems" approach/"problem-based", etc.? Are computers used in the coursework?

27. Will the school's curriculum change in any way next year (or the next few years)?

28. Are there summer courses at this school?

29. Are there summer programs (clinical or research) available at this school?

30. Could you tell me about the hospitals where students do their clinical rotations?

31. Are there other clinical settings where students rotate (*e.g.* doctors' offices, rural clinics, ambulatory medical or surgical centers, inner city clinics, etc.)?

32. What types of research opportunities are available for students? How often do they get published?

33. Does your school have specific scholarships that I can apply for? How do I find out about them?

34. Does the school's financial aid office provide short-term loans or "emergency" loans to students?

35. Do you anticipate an increase in your tuition and fees? How much of an increase? Will these costs stabilize or will there be further increases over the next few years?

36. What student organizations are available to join in the medical school?

37 What do medical students do socially? What are the advantages to this geographic area?

38. Do students involve themselves in community service?

39. How successful are students' spouses in finding employment in the community or with the university system?

40. How often are exams?

41. Is a note-taking service provided for the students? Is it for all/some of the courses? Does the medical school operate the service or do students run it? What is the cost for the student?

42. Is on-campus housing available for single students? . . . for married students or for those with children?

43. What is the policy for students sitting on different medical school committees? For example, can medical students serve on the admissions committee? How many serve in this capacity? How do they obtain these positions?—elected or appointed?

44. How long are your exams? Are there "exam blocks" during the first year? (Tests are given during a "final exam week" type arrangement.) How often do these blocks occur?

45. Is there an Honors Code System at your school?

46. If a student has a formal complaint or grievance, is there a formal appeals process? How does it work?

47. What are the procedures/protocols for students who get exposed to an infectious disease (*e.g.* a needle-stick accident)?

48. Is disability insurance available for students?

49. Do students have cars when doing their clinical rotations? Are there any parking problems or safety issues?

50. If you had the opportunity to choose any medical school again, would you come here? Why/why not?

Know About the Medical School's Curriculum

There are a few basic approaches to medical education in the United States:

1   THE TRADITIONAL MEDICAL SCHOOL DISCIPLINE APPROACH.

Many schools utilize this traditional method of education: a combination of lectures/labs for each of the separate basic medical science disciplines (*e.g.* anatomy, biochemistry, physiology, histology, pharmacology, pathology, etc.).

2.   THE SYSTEMS APPROACH.

Study of the human body is accomplished by examining each of the systems/regions (*e.g.* cardiovascular, endocrine, reproductive, immune, renal, gastrointestinal, etc.) and learning their anatomy, histology, physiology, etc. through an interdisciplinary approach. Students do not take separate courses in each of the basic medical science disciplines as in the first approach.

3.   PROBLEM-BASED LEARNING.

Small groups of five to seven students meet with faculty members who "facilitate" learning through a discussion of problem-oriented/clinical cases. Course objectives are set up by the appropriate departments and there is an emphasis on student "self-directed" learning.

A number of medical schools will combine one or more approaches, whereas at some schools there will be one dominant approach. No matter what curriculum approach is used, a variety of educational methods will be provided during your basic medical science years; examples include lectures, labs, small group discussions/tutorials, seminars, computer-assisted learning, and clinical simulations/demonstrations.

(NOTE: The Association of American Medical Colleges (AAMC) publishes the AAMC Curriculum Directory which is an excellent source regarding a medical school's curriculum.)

Other Important Areas That You May Need to Address

1.   APPLICANTS WITHOUT AN IN-STATE MEDICAL SCHOOL. (There are various state programs that provide opportunities for those applicants.)

If you are a resident of one of these states (*e.g.* Alaska, Montana, Wyoming, Idaho, Maine) you must make sure that you meet the requirements and follow all the guidelines of the various state programs. The opportunity to attend a medical school will depend on funding/contractual agreements between these states and certain medical schools. Two of these opportunities—the Western Interstate Commission for Higher Education (WICHE) Professional Student Exchange Program and the WAMI (Washington, Alaska, Montana, Idaho) Program are discussed in Chapter 12, "The Medical School Application Process." The WICHE Professional Student Exchange Program (for allopathic medical schools) involves the states of Alaska, Montana, and Wyoming and medical schools in Arizona, California, Colorado, Hawaii, Nevada, New Mexico, North Dakota, Oregon, and Utah. Under the WICHE Program, students from Alaska, Hawaii, Montana, Wyoming, and other western states may also attend the Western University of Health Sciences/College of Osteopathic Medicine of the Pacific. The WAMI Program involves the University of Washington School of Medicine and the states of Montana, Alaska, and Idaho. Note that if you are a resident of Maine, the University of Vermont College of Medicine has a contractual agreement with your state.

Remember that the funding, contractual agreements and requirements/guidelines can change in any given year, so it is important to update yourself on these programs.

2. EARLY DECISION PROGRAM (EDP)

This is a unique opportunity to apply to one medical school early in the application process. To apply as an EDP candidate, you should have excellent credentials and have a strong desire to attend that school where you are applying. If you are accepted, you must attend that school; if you are not accepted, you will still have sufficient time to apply to other medical schools. The Early Decision Program is discussed in Chapter 12, "The Medical School Application Process."

3. DEFERRED ENTRANCE INTO MEDICAL SCHOOL

Many medical schools will accept requests for deferred entrance (one-year) into their accepted first year class. Of these medical schools, most will require the accepted student to put his/her request in writing with an explanation of the reason(s) for the deferment. There is a variety of reasons for requesting a deferment: personal, employment/financial, research, travel, etc. These deferment requests are then examined on an individual basis by the medical school.

4. ENRICHMENT PROGRAMS

Some medical schools will offer summer programs for students entering the first year class. They are designed to introduce the student to the curriculum and the academic expectations in medical school. These programs usually have lectures/laboratory work in one or more basic medical science areas. Many times there are also other opportunities provided for the students which will help them when they begin their first semester;

examples include seminars on study skills and basic medical science course learning strategies. The form of these programs may vary: students may receive an overview of the first year basic science curriculum or may concentrate on one course. (NOTE: Whether or not a student receives academic credit for the summer program also depends on the school. Enrollment numbers in these programs will depend on the individual medical school and the availability of funding.)

5. FLEXIBLE/DECELERATED/ALTERNATE SCHEDULING

Some medical schools offer students the opportunity to fulfill their academic requirements over a five year period. These programs may involve summer coursework and/or extending the first or second year of medical school over a period of two years.

6. ACCELERATED PROGRAMS

Besides the six or seven year B.S. - B.A./M.D. programs, there are some medical schools that allow students to complete the four year curriculum in three years. (These students usually have very strong science backgrounds.)

17
Statistics for Premedical Students

Premedical students realize that their hard work is "not done in a vacuum"—results and accomplishments are measured in terms of gaining admission into medical school. At the same time, however, "numbers" do not always translate into individual choices regarding premedical course planning and medical school application strategies. To choose a major, for example, based on its success of gaining admission into medical school, may translate into a decision that does not coincide with one's interests.

Statistical information does help the student understand "trends" in the application process—it is now, for example, becoming more difficult to obtain admission into medical school based on the number of applicants. The following information in this chapter was collected by the Association of American Medical Colleges (AAMC) and published in its book, *Medical School Admission Requirements, United States and Canada 1998-1999.*

I am using sections from various tables with the permission of the Association of American Medical Colleges.

I have used informational excerpts from the following general areas:

1. Course Requirements For Medical School Admission (1998-1999 Entering Class).

2. Acceptance Into Medical School by Undergraduate Major (1996-1997 Entering Class).

3. Application Trends For First Year Entering Classes.

4. Acceptance Information For Male and Female Applicants.

5. Acceptance Rates by Age/Sex of the 1996-1997 Entering Class.

6. Minority Group Application/Acceptance Information.

7. Additional Information For Female Applicants.

Table 1
**Courses Required by 10 or More Medical Schools (U.S.)
for the 1998-1999 Entering Class**

Required Subject	No. of Schools *(n=118)
Physics	117
Organic chemistry	117
Inorganic (general) chemistry	115
English	80
Biology	66
Biology or zoology	54
Calculus	24
College mathematics	22

* Seven out of the 125 medical schools did not indicate specific course requirements and were not included in this data.

NOTE: A smaller number of schools also require subjects such as humanities, behavioral and/or social sciences.

(Source: Association of American Medical Colleges (AAMC), *Medical School Admission Requirements (MSAR), United States and Canada 1998-1999,* p. 22.)

Table 2
Undergraduate Majors and Acceptance to Medical School
(1996-1997 Entering Class)

Undergraduate Major	Total Applicants		Accepted Applicants	
	No.	% of Total	No.	% of Major
Biological Sciences				
Biology	17,713	37.7	6,163	34.8
Microbiology	1,092	2.3	357	32.7
Zoology	1,073	2.3	349	32.5
Physical Sciences				
Biochemistry	2,732	5.8	1,160	42.5
Chemical Engineering	494	1.1	203	41.1
Chemistry	2,709	5.8	1,049	38.7
Electrical Engineering	483	1.0	184	38.1
Mathematics	322	.7	135	41.9
Physics	300	.6	127	42.3
Nonscience Subjects				
Economics	493	1.0	205	41.6
English	734	1.6	337	45.9
Foreign Language	387	.8	154	39.8
History	597	1.3	295	49.4
Philosophy	228	.5	114	50.0
Political Science	370	.8	154	41.6
Psychology	2,507	5.3	856	34.1
Sociology	202	.4	72	35.6
Other Health Professions				
Nursing	316	.7	53	16.8
Pharmacy	317	.7	83	26.2
Mixed Disciplines				
Double Major Science	824	1.8	311	37.7
Double Major Non-Science	1,188	2.5	504	42.4

(Association of American Medical Colleges, *Medical School Admission Requirements, United States and Canada 1998-1999,* p. 24.)

Table 3
Application Trends for First Year Entering Classes

Entering Year	Individuals Filing Applications	Applications Filed	Number of New Entrants*	Percent of Applicants Enrolled
1994-95	45,365	561,593	16,287	36
1995-96	46,591	595,975	16,253	35
1996-97	46,968	566,122	16,200	35

NOTE: In 1992-1993 there were 37,410 individuals filing applications with 44 percent of the applicants enrolled.

* New entrants are students entering medical school for the first time.

(Association of American Medical Colleges, *Medical School Admission Requirements, United States and Canada 1998-1999,* p. 46.)

Table 4
Acceptance Information for Male and Female Applicants

First Year Class	No. of Applicants		No. Accepted		% Accepted	
	Men	Women	Men	Women	Men	Women
1994-95	26,397	18,968	10,062	7,255	38.1	38.2
1995-96	26,812	19,779	9,920	7,437	37.0	37.6
1996-97	26,937	20,031	9,946	7,439	36.9	37.1

(Association of American Medical Colleges, *Medical School Admission Requirements, United States and Canada 1998-1999,* p. 36 .)

Table 5
Acceptance Rates by Age and Sex of the 1996-1997 Entering Class

| | Men | | | Women | | |
Age	No. of Applicants	Percent	Percent Accepted	No. of Applicants	Percent	Percent Accepted
20 and under	403	1.5	68.2	368	1.8	64.1
21-23	13,531	50.2	44.9	10,792	53.9	43.7
24-27	8,322	30.9	29.0	5,583	27.9	30.1
28-31	2,603	9.7	27.4	1,671	8.3	26.4
32-34	922	3.4	25.6	634	3.2	25.4
35-37	573	2.1	21.1	428	2.1	23.6
38 and over	583	2.2	18.2	555	2.8	19.5

(Association of American Medical Colleges, *Medical School Admission Requirements, United States and Canada 1998-1999,* p. 35.)

Table 6
Minority Group Application And Acceptance Information

| | Black American | | | | American Indian | | | |
| | Applicants | | Acceptees | | Applicants | | Acceptees | |
First Year Class	No.	% of All Applicants	No.	% Accepted	No.	% of All Applicants	No.	% Accepted
1994-95	3,659	8.1	1,427	39.0	261	0.6	116	44.4
1995-96	3,595	7.7	1,407	39.1	305	0.7	138	45.2
1996-97	3,645	7.7	1,305	35.8	323	0.7	134	41.5

| | Mexican American/Chicano | | | | Mainland Puerto Rican | | | |
| | Applicants | | Acceptees | | Applicants | | Acceptees | |
First Year Class	No.	% of All Applicants	No.	% Accepted	No.	% of All Applicants	No.	% Accepted
1994-95	861	1.9	478	55.5	279	0.6	152	54.5
1995-96	917	2.0	497	54.2	329	0.7	137	41.6
1996-97	964	2.1	466	48.3	327	0.7	165	50.5

(Association of American Medical Colleges, *Medical School Admission Requirements, United States and Canada 1998-1999,* p. 36.)

Table 7
Female Applicants and First-Year Women
New Entrants to Medical School (U.S.)

First Year Class	Total Applicants	Women Applicants	% of Total Applicants	Total First-Year New Entrants*	Women First-Year New Entrants	% of Total First-Year New Entrants*
1994-95	45,365	18,968	41.8	16,287	6,819	41.9
1995-96	46,591	19,779	42.5	16,253	6,941	42.7
1996-97	46,968	20,031	42.6	16,200	6,917	42.7

* First-year new entrants are those students entering medical school for the first time.

(Association of American Medical Colleges, *Medical School Admission Requirements, United States and Canada 1998-1999,* p. 35)

18

Specialized Graduate and Professional School Joint Programs

As the world around us has become a complex place, so too has the practice of medicine. Health care has become increasingly intertwined with other professions including law, business, public health, and public policy. The practice of medicine is becoming extremely diverse. Universities across the nation have responded to the need and demand for "cross-discipline" educated physicians. There are now a myriad of opportunities for students to combine their medical training with their other interests.

Listed below are examples of combined degree ("joint degree") programs which are available to medical school applicants. (The applicant will still need to apply separately to each school for admission.) There are also many medical schools which also allow the student to apply for admission to the other part of the "joint program" (*e.g.* M.B.A., M.P.H., etc.) once they are already matriculated.

1. M.D./Ph.D.-Medical Scientist Training Program (MSTP)

This is a very highly selective program that is sponsored by the National Institutes of Health (NIH). It provides financial support (yearly tuition and stipend) for highly qualified students who seek potential careers in research/academic medicine. Though this program is limited to six years of support, many students may require seven or more years to complete their M.D./Ph.D.'s (exclusive of residency). Most medical schools then seek their own financial sources for the M.D./Ph.D.-MSTP candidate to finish his/her studies. A wide variety of medical science disciplines are available and depend on the individual university's program. There are currently (1997-1998) about 150 new admittees each year with a total of 33 medical schools receiving MSTP grant money. (An address for additional information about this program is provided on the following page. A list of 1997 MSTP programs is also given. The medical school list may change in any given application year so it is important to update your information for that year.)

For additional information, the following contact address is provided:

Medical Scientist Training Program (MSTP)
National Institutes of Health
45 Center Drive, MSC 6200
Bethesda, MD 20892-6200
(301) 594-3830

M.D./Ph.D.-Medical Scientist Training Program (MSTP) 1997 Programs: (This list is provided by the National Institutes of Health.)

Medical Schools

Alabama

University of Alabama

California

Stanford

UCLA

University of California,   San Diego

University of California, San Francisco

Colorado

University of Colorado

Connecticut

Yale University

Georgia

Emory University

Illinois

University of Chicago

Northwestern University

Iowa

University of Iowa

Maryland

Johns Hopkins

Massachusetts

Harvard

Tufts

Michigan

University of Michigan

Minnesota

University of Minnesota
(Minneapolis)

Missouri

Washington University
(St. Louis)

New York

Albert Einstein

Columbia University

Cornell University

Mount Sinai

New York University

University of Rochester

SUNY-Stony Brook

North Carolina

Duke

Ohio

Case Western Reserve

Pennsylvania

University of Pennsylvania

University of Pittsburgh

Tennessee

Vanderbilt University

Texas

Baylor

University of Texas, Dallas

(Southwestern)

Virginia

University of Virginia

Washington

University of Washington

2. M.D./Ph.D. (Medical/Graduate School Sponsored)

There are well over 100 medical schools that provide funding support for their own joint programs. The number of areas (*e.g.* Biochemistry, Pharmacology, Physiology, etc.) are quite varied depending on the individual school. Some universities also offer opportunities to pursue a Ph.D. in a non-science discipline. The AAMC publishes the yearly book, *Medical School Admission Requirements*. This resource provides both contact addresses regarding M.D./Ph.D. programs and also has a comprehensive table of medical science disciplines offered at the numerous schools. To seek information about non-science Ph.D.'s, the applicant will need to write to individual schools about their availability.

3. MEDICINE AND PUBLIC HEALTH (M.D./M.P.H.) Master of Public Health

Preventive medicine, health promotion, environmental, and occupational health are just some of the important areas involved in public health.

M.D./M.P.H. Programs

University of Arizona

University of California, Davis

University of California, San Francisco

George Washington University

University of South Florida

Emory University

Morehouse School of Medicine

Northwestern University

Tulane University

Boston University

Harvard University

Tufts University

University of Michigan

Saint Louis University

Duke University

UMDNJ-Robert Wood Johnson
    Medical School

Columbia University

University of North Carolina-Chapel Hill

Oregon Health Sciences University

Jefferson Medical College of
    Thomas Jefferson University

University of South Carolina

4. MEDICINE AND BUSINESS (M.D./M.B.A., Master of Business Administration)

Mergers/acquisitions/consolidations. . . HMO's/PPO's. . . The future of American medicine has already arrived!

M.D./M.B.A. Programs

University of California, Davis

University of California, Irvine

Georgetown University

University of Chicago

University of Illinois

Northwestern University
(M.D./M.M., Master of Management)

Tufts University

Dartmouth

Duke

Jefferson National College of Thomas
    Jefferson University

5. MEDICINE AND LAW (M.D./J.D., Juris Doctorate)

   Medical ethics/risk management/health care legislation/medical malpractice— all of these issues, along with other medical/legal aspects, impact directly on medicine.

M.D./J.D. Programs

Yale

University of Chicago

University of Illinois

Southern Illinois

UMDNJ-Robert Wood Johnson Medical School (with Rutgers Law School)

Duke

University of North Carolina, Chapel Hill

6. MEDICINE AND PUBLIC POLICY (M.D./M.P.P., Master of Public Policy)

   Harvard   Duke

7. MEDICAL HISTORY (M.D./M.A. or M.D./Ph.D.)

   Duke

8. MEDICINE AND THEOLOGY (M.D./M.Div., Master of Divinity)

   Yale

Though the above list is detailed, it cannot list every possible combination. Some schools will allow the student to pursue a M.S. or Ph.D. degree in an area outside of the medical sciences. Students have even been able to obtain advanced degrees in engineering. The offerings of such programs can change on a yearly basis; the best resource will be the schools themselves—make sure you read the current catalogs/brochures for that application year.

It will be necessary, of course, for the applicant to be accepted by both schools. You will also need to fulfill the other program's application requirements (*e.g.* taking the Graduate Management Admissions Test [GMAT] for an M.B.A.), independent from those of medical school. Depending on the university, some joint programs may also involve summer courses. If you are interested in such opportunities, it will be important to know both the academic year schedules and the time periods involved. The M.D./M.B.A., for example, usually takes five years to complete. If you studied for each degree separately, it would take six years. You need to remember the other factors involved in such a commitment: length of program, financial cost, and perhaps the lack of a guaranteed "perfect job" for your credentials.

When you apply for a joint program, you must also have appropriate reasons for seeking the additional education. Admission committees know that medical school is, in itself, a very difficult professional program. They will definitely want to know about your interests and motivations and their potential impact on your future personal and professional life.

19

Combined Bachelor Degree/M.D. Programs Early Assurance Programs

High School and College Applicants

If you are a high school senior with top grades and SAT/ACT scores and are seeking a medical career, you may be a potential applicant for one of the unique BS or BA/M.D. combined programs. There are basically two types of programs—the accelerated six or seven-year bachelor degree/M.D. curriculum or the non-accelerated combined eight-year program. These degree programs will assure you a spot in a medical school class—you are "provisionally admitted" into medical school as a high school senior, but you must first complete your undergraduate years (with acceptable academic credentials). The completion of your undergraduate program will take two or three years (accelerated programs) or four years (non-accelerated). The student then enters medical school for the regular four-year curriculum of basic medical science and clinical clerkships.

There are also some "Early Assurance" Programs which have the student apply for an "assured medical school position" while he/she is an undergraduate. As with the high school applicants, these college undergraduates are "provisionally admitted" into medical school. Though most of these schools require the student to finish four years of college, there are some programs that are accelerated.

At the end of this chapter is a list of school addresses along with some of the highlights from each program. Be aware that every Combined Bachelor Degree/M.D. Program or Early Assurance Program will have their own admission requirements. Each school will also require the student to achieve certain objective criteria (GPA and MCAT, if appropriate) and maintain professional behavior as prerequisites to formal admission.

Listed below are some of the factors to consider when applying and/or enrolling in a Combined Bachelor Degree/M.D. or an Early Assurance Program:

1. If you apply as a high school senior, the acceptance into such programs usually requires "all-star" student status. Depending on the program, the SAT score averages usually range between 1100 and 1500. Many programs are in the 1300-1400 range (some programs also

accept ACT scores). Class rank is also very important. Most programs will expect you to be in the top 5-10 percent of your high school class. Some programs have even stricter requirements (top 2-3 percent) while a few require you to be in the top 20 percent.

2. Each school will require you to have a strong foundation in English, math, foreign language, natural sciences, and humanities.

3. Your motivation and desire to enter medicine at an early age will also be examined carefully. Committees want to make sure that it is YOUR DECISION and not that of your parents, relatives, or friends. Your interest in medicine should also be evidenced by a health care related work experience (paid or volunteer: hospital or clinical work or having a preceptorship with a physician).

4. Be aware that some schools may limit their programs to state residents or have a "strong preference for state residents."

5. With the goal of having more "broadly educated" physicians, more programs are emphasizing additional liberal arts requirements in the social sciences and humanities. Most programs also emphasize that you can major in a non-science. Some schools also give students the option to "extend" the time duration of their program so that they can take full advantage of taking additional non-science courses.

6. You will still complete all premedical requirements for that medical school. Six-year programs will usually require you to take courses one or two summers while registered as an undergraduate.

7. "Entering class" sizes may vary on a yearly basis depending on the quality of the applicant pool. There is usually a maximum number of positions the program can fill—in any given year, however, all positions may not be filled.

8. Many programs will have organized clinical externships/preceptorships for their students while they are undergraduates. Some programs will also offer research opportunities.

9. Interviews for such programs usually occur with the undergraduate institution, the medical school, and/or a joint committee of the undergraduate/medical school. A student may also be interviewed after he/she has completed one or more years in the undergraduate program.

10. Some eight-year programs will only grant you admission after you have completed two to three years of coursework and have taken the MCATs.

11. Most medical schools in accelerated/non-accelerated BS-BA/M.D. programs will require the MCAT.

12. Admitted applicants are expected to exhibit leadership, maturity, and personal qualities suitable for a career in medicine.

13. Having a provisional, guaranteed spot in medical school removes inordinate amounts of

stress and anxiety; achieve and maintain at least the minimum requirements—and you're in! Some programs remove even more stress by not requiring the MCAT!

14. If you later intend to apply to other medical schools, you will lose your guaranteed/provisional first year position in the present medical school.

15. Have a FINANCIAL PLAN. When you get accepted into such a program, you are looking at financing your next six to eight years. Many programs involve private undergraduate institutions/private medical schools—the total cost will be quite substantial compared to a state university medical school.

Combined Bachelor Degree/M.D. Programs
Early Assurance Programs

(Programs marked with an asterisk (*) require the student to apply for early acceptance as a college undergraduate [not as a high school senior].)

This section has the following information:

1. Accelerated (less than 8 years) and Non-Accelerated (8 years) Bachelor Degree/M.D. Programs and Early Assurance Programs

2. Addresses of all programs are listed at the end of the chapter. With many programs, the initial inquiries are made through the undergraduate institution.

3. Addresses of all United States Allopathic (M.D.) medical schools are listed in Appendix A.

4. While many programs require the student to apply as a high school senior, there are some that accept applications only after the student is in college for a certain time period. An asterisk (*) indicates these programs where the student applies for early acceptance while enrolled as an undergraduate.

5. There is also an overview of the programs and depending on the availability of information, the descriptions may include the following: time length of program, SAT/ACT scores, research and externship/preceptorship activities, course offerings, types of majors, entering class size, appropriate time for applying (if it is a program which requires students to apply as undergraduates), residency requirements, and other opportunities (*e.g.* minority students, rural health care, primary care medicine).

6. Requirements and program descriptions may change. The applicant should keep himself/herself updated on such information before formally applying to a program(s).

Accelerated Programs

Under this heading you will find Combined Bachelor Degree/M.D. or Early Assurance Programs with the following time periods of completion:

1. 6-year programs

2. 6-year programs (with 7th year optional)

3. 7-year programs

4. 7-year programs (with 8th year optional)

CALIFORNIA

University of California, Riverside/University of California, Los Angeles UCLA School of Medicine

1. 7-year program.

2. Biomedical sciences major with broad exposure to the social sciences and humanities.

3. First five years at UCLA Riverside—includes the first two years of basic medical science courses of medical school.The student attends the UCLA School of Medicine for the last two years (clinical rotations).

4. Average SAT score: greater than 1200.

5. Entering class: up to 24.

6. Out-of-state residents are eligible to apply.

DISTRICT OF COLUMBIA

Howard University College of Liberal Arts/Howard University College of Medicine

1. 6-year program.

2. Liberal arts education is emphasized.

3. Students can major in a science or a non-science discipline.

4. Average SAT score: 1300; average ACT score: range 25-29.

5. Entering class: up to 10.

6. Out-of-state residents are eligible to apply.

*Howard University College of Medicine Early Entry Medical Education Program (EEMEP)

Early Entry Medical Education Program

1. 7-year program.
2. The student must complete 62 credit hours of college coursework (including premedical courses) in order to apply.
3. Applicant must attend an accredited four-year college or university.
4. Out-of-state residents are eligible to apply.

George Washington University/George Washington University School of Medicine

1. 7-year program.
2. Students can major in a science or a non-science discipline.
3. Average SAT score: 1450; average ACT score: 32.
4. Entering class: up to 10.
5. Out-of-state residents are eligible to apply.

FLORIDA

*University of Florida College of Medicine Junior Honors Medical Program

Junior Honors Medical Program

1. 7-year program.
2. Students apply during their sophomore year in college.
3. Students can major in a science or a non-science discipline.
4. Basic medical science seminars are offered on the undergraduate level.
5. The program is intended primarily for University of Florida students. Applications from students at other colleges/universities may be considered.
6. Entering class: maximum of 12.
7. Preference is given to Florida residents.

<u>University of Miami/University of Miami School of Medicine</u>

1. 6 or 7-year option.

2. Minimum SAT score: 1360; ACT score: 31.

3. Biology/Chemistry/Physics majors are most popular.

4. Undergraduate research opportunities.

5. Entering class: up to 20.

6. Only Florida residents may apply to this program.

ILLINOIS

<u>Northwestern University/Northwestern University Medical School</u>

1. 7-year program.

2. Students can major in a science or a non-science discipline.

3. Average SAT score: over 1500.

4. Entering class: up to 60 students.

5. Out-of-state residents are eligible to apply.

MASSACHUSETTS

<u>Boston University College of Arts and Sciences/Boston University School of Medicine</u>

1. 7-year program (8-year option).

2. Humanities and social science courses are offered.

3. Average SAT score: 1500.

4. Entering class: up to 25.

5. Out-of-state residents are eligible to apply.

MISSOURI

<u>University of Missouri, Kansas City (UMKC) College of Arts and Sciences or the UMKC School of Biological Sciences/UMKC School of Medicine</u>

1. 6-year program.
2. Liberal arts are emphasized.
3. Students can major in a science or a non-science discipline.
4. Early exposure to clinical medicine.
5. Entering class: up to 100.
6. Out-of-state residents are eligible to apply.

NEBRASKA

Chadron State College/University of Nebraska Medical Center, University of Nebraska College of Medicine

Rural Health Opportunities Program (RHOP)

1. 7-year program.
2. Commitment to practicing as a physician in the rural areas of Nebraska.
3. Entering class: up to 5.
4. Eligibility: Rural Nebraska students.

Wayne State College/University of Nebraska Medical Center, University of Nebraska College of Medicine

Rural Health Opportunities Program (RHOP)

1. 7-year program.
2. Commitment to practicing as a physician in the rural areas of Nebraska.
3. Entering class: up to 5.
4. Eligibility: Rural Nebraska students.

NEW JERSEY

UMDNJ-New Jersey Medical School (The New Jersey Medical School of the University of Medicine and Dentistry of New Jersey)

1. 7-year program in affiliation with the following seven undergraduate institutions (addresses available at the end of this chapter):

   - Drew University (NJ)
   - Montclair State University (NJ)
   - New Jersey Institute of Technology
   - Stevens Institute of Technology (NJ)
   - The Richard Stockton College of New Jersey
   - The College of New Jersey
   - Boston University (MA) (Program is only for NJ residents)

2. Variety of majors (including engineering) depending upon the undergraduate institution.

3. Average minimum SAT scores: 1350-1400.

4. Out-of-state residents are eligible to apply.

5. Entering class: up to 25 students (total number).

6. The Boston University/UMDNJ-New Jersey Medical School Program is limited to New Jersey residents attending Boston University.

*The Richard Stockton College of New Jersey/University of Medicine and Dentistry of New Jersey (UMDNJ) - Robert Wood Johnson Medical School

1. 7-year program (8-year option).

2. Students can major in a science or a non-science discipline.

3. Application process can begin at the end of the sophomore year.

4. Entering class: No set number.

5. Out-of-state residents are eligible to apply.

NEW YORK

Rensselaer Polytechnic Institute/Albany Medical College

1. 6-year program.

2. Average SAT score: 1450.

3. Entering class: up to 20.

4. Out-of-state residents are eligible to apply.

Sophie Davis School of Biomedical Education, City University of New York (CUNY)/ affiliated with seven New York State medical schools

1. 7-year program.

2. Purposes of this program are to increase the number of primary care doctors working in under-served urban settings and to increase minority physician numbers.

3. Average SAT score: greater than 1200.

4. Three years of college and two basic medical science years are spent at CUNY. Students then transfer to a participating medical school for their clinical training (last two years).

5. Entering class: 60.

6. New York State residents are only eligible to apply.

Union College/Albany Medical College

1. 7-year program.

2. Allowance for a broad-based education in the social sciences/humanities.

3. Average SAT score: 1300 or higher.

4. Entering class: up to 20.

5. Out-of-state residents are eligible to apply.

OHIO

University of Akron, Kent State University, Youngstown State University/Northeastern Ohio Universities College of Medicine (NEOUCOM)

1. 6 or 7-year program.

2. Must attend one of the following three universities:
    - University of Akron
    - Kent State University
    - Youngstown State University

3. Strong preference is given to Ohio residents.

4. Average SAT score: greater than 1300; average ACT score: 30.

5. Entering class: 105

6. Out-of-state residents are eligible to apply.

PENNSYLVANIA

*Duquesne University/Allegheny University of the Health Sciences: Medical College of Pennsylvania/Hahnemann School of Medicine

1. 7-year program.

2. Students can major in a science or a non-science discipline.

3. Students apply in the second semester of their sophomore year in college.

4. Hospital and/or physician preceptorships are offered.

5. Entering class: up to 6.

6. Out-of-state residents are eligible to apply.

Lehigh University/Allegheny University of the Health Sciences: Medical College of Pennsylvania/Hahnemann School of Medicine

1. 6-year program (optional 7-year program).

2. Minimum SAT score: 1360.

3. Entering class: up to 10 per year.

4. Out-of-state residents are eligible to apply.

Pennsylvania State University/Jefferson Medical College of Thomas Jefferson University

1. 6-year program.

2. Minimum SAT score: 1380.

3. Entering class: average is 30 students.

4. Pennsylvania residents are given preference but out-of-state applicants are eligible to apply.

Villanova University/Allegheny University of the Health Sciences: Medical College of Pennsylvania/Hahnemann School of Medicine

1. 6 or 7-year program.

2. Majors: Biology or a Bachelor of Science Comprehensive (BSC) major. BSC emphasizes physics and mathematics.

3. Minimum SAT score: 1360; average ACT score: 31.

4. Entering class: average 20 to 30.

5. Out-of-state residents are eligible to apply.

West Chester University/Allegheny University of the Health Sciences: Medical College of Pennsylvania/Hahnemann School of Medicine

1. 7-year program.

2. SAT standard: 1370.

3. Biomedical research internships are available for full credit (junior year).

4. Entering class: up to 5.

5. Out-of-state residents are eligible to apply.

TENNESSEE

*Fisk University/Meharry Medical College

1. 7-year program.

2. Students are selected after their first undergraduate semester. Preference is given to minority applicants.

3. SAT/ACT scores/high school rank is considered.

4. Entering class: up to 12.

5. Out-of-state residents are eligible to apply.

WISCONSIN

University of Wisconsin-Madison/University of Wisconsin Medical School

1. 7-year program (8 to 9-year option).

2. Students can major in a science or a non-science discipline.

3. Minimum SAT score: 1300; ACT score: 30.

4. Entering class: maximum of 50.

5. Admission is limited to Wisconsin residents.

Non-Accelerated Combined Bachelor Degree/M.D. Programs or Early Assurance Programs (8 Years)

ALABAMA

University of Alabama at Birmingham (UAB)/University of Alabama School of Medicine

Early Medical School Acceptance Program (EMSAP)

1. 8-year program.

2. Students can major in a science or a non-science discipline.

3. Medical related experiences are provided for students as undergraduates.

4. Entering class: up to 10.

5. Preference is given to Alabama residents.

University of South Alabama/University of South Alabama College of Medicine

1. 8-year program.

2. Minimum ACT score: 28 (or comparable SAT score)

3. Entering class: 15-19.

4. Out-of-state residents are eligible to apply.

CALIFORNIA

University of Southern California College of Letters, Arts, and Sciences/University of Southern California School of Medicine

1. 8-year program.

2. A broad education in the liberal arts is encouraged.

3. Students can major in a science or a non-science discipline.

4. Volunteer opportunities.

5. Average SAT score: over 1450.

6. Entering class: 35.

7. Out-of-state residents are eligible to apply.

DELAWARE

*University of Delaware (Medical Scholars Program)/Jefferson Medical College of Thomas Jefferson University

1. 8-year program.

2. Students can major in a science or a non-science discipline.

3. Apply for the Combined Bachelor Degree/M.D. program during the freshman or sopho-more year (conditional acceptance).

4. Must complete at least 55 credit hours of Life and Physical Sciences.

5. Broad spectrum of liberal arts courses are offered.

6. Entering class: maximum of 15.

7. Out-of-state residents attending the University of Delaware are eligible to apply.

The Delaware Institute of Medical Education and Research (DIMER) Program/Jefferson Medical College of Thomas Jefferson University

1. 8-year program.

2. Students can major in a science or a non-science discipline.

3. Students can attend any four year accredited college/university in the United States or Canada.

4. A minimum of 20 positions are available every year for qualified candidates.

5. Open only to Delaware residents.

DISTRICT OF COLUMBIA

*George Washington University/George Washington University School of Medicine and Health Sciences

The Early Selection Program

1. 8-year program.
2. Students apply during their sophomore year in college.
3. Students can major in a science or a non-science discipline.
4. Entering class: up to 15.
5. Out-of-state residents are eligible to apply.

*Georgetown University/Georgetown University School of Medicine

Early Assurance Program

1. 8-year program.
2. Students can major in a science or a non-science discipline.
3. Students apply at the end of their sophomore year.
4. Entering class: no established acceptance allotment.
5. Out-of-state residents are eligible to apply.

ILLINOIS

Illinois Institute of Technology/Finch University of Health Sciences-Chicago Medical School

1. 8-year program.
2. Majors: chemical, mechanical, or electrical engineering or computer science.
3. Average SAT score: approximately 1300.
4. Entering class: up to 15.
5. Out-of-state residents are eligible to apply.

MASSACHUSETTS

*Boston University/Boston University School of Medicine

MMEDIC Program: Modular Medical Integrated Curriculum

1. 8-year program.
2. Offered through the College of Liberal Arts and the Boston University School of Medicine.
3. Various electives in the social sciences and humanities.
4. Apply during sophomore year; accepted candidates finish their junior and senior year before beginning medical school.
5. Modular courses are also offered during the junior and senior year. These courses are some of the same basic science disciplines taken during the first year of medical school.
6. Available positions: up to 15.
7. Out-of-state residents are eligible to apply.

*Boston University/Boston University School of Medicine

ENGMEDIC Program: Engineering/Medical Integrated Curriculum

1. 8-year program.
2. The undergraduate part of the program is in the Department of Biomedical Engineering (B.S. in Biomedical Engineering).
3. Apply during sophomore year; accepted candidates finish their junior and senior year before beginning medical school.
4. Available positions: up to 5.
5. Out-of-state residents are eligible to apply.

Boston University School of Medicine/Early Medical School Selection Program (EMSSP)

Early Medical School Selection Program (EMSSP)

1. 8-year program.
2. Developed with a group of historically black colleges and universities. Also includes students from colleges/universities with large Hispanic populations and the Indian Health Service.
3. First three years are spent at the students' respective colleges/universities. Senior year is spent at Boston University.

*Brandeis University/Mt. Sinai School of Medicine

1. 8-year program.
2. Non-science majors only.
3. Apply for early acceptance during the sophomore year.
4. Summer programs (after junior year) at Mt. Sinai School of Medicine.
5. Entering class: up to 5.
6. Out-of-state residents are eligible to apply.

*Brandeis University/Tufts University School of Medicine

1. 8-year program.
2. Choice of majors (science or non-science).
3. Apply for early acceptance in the sophomore year.
4. Entering class: up to 5.
5. Out-of-state residents are eligible to apply.

MICHIGAN

University of Michigan College of Literature, Science, and Arts/University of Michigan Medical School

1. 8-year program.
2. Liberal arts curriculum. Students can major in a science or a non-science discipline.
3. First year clinical preceptorship.
4. Average SAT score: greater than 1350; average ACT score: 31.
5. Entering class: up to 40.
6. Out-of-state residents are eligible to apply.

Michigan State University/Michigan State University College of Human Medicine

1. 8-year program.
2. Liberal arts are emphasized. Students can major in a science or a non-science discipline.

3. Physician mentorship program.

4. Research experience provided.

5. SAT score: 1280; ACT score: 29.

6. Entering class: up to 10.

7. Out-of-state residents are eligible to apply.

NEW JERSEY

Monmouth University/Allegheny University of the Health Sciences: Medical College of Pennsylvania/Hahnemann School of Medicine

1. 8-year program.

2. Minimum SAT score: 1270 (no score lower than 560).

3. Students can major in a science or a non-science discipline.

4. Hospital preceptorship during senior year.

5. Entering class: up to 4.

6. Preference is given to New Jersey and Delaware residents.

*Rutgers University/University of Medicine and Dentistry of New Jersey UMDNJ—Robert Wood Johnson Medical School

1. 8-year program.

2. Liberal arts courses are encouraged.

3. Average SAT score: greater than 1300.

4. Students are chosen at the end of their sophomore year in college. The student's high school record is also a factor for admission.

5. Students must be attending Rutgers University.

6. Entering class: 12-15.

7. Out-of-state residents are eligible to apply.

NEW YORK

Binghamton University/State University of New York (SUNY) Health Science Center at Syracuse College of Medicine

1. 8-year program.
2. Resident of a New York State rural area.
3. Interest in a primary care specialty (family practice, general internal medicine, or general pediatrics) in a physician under-served area.
4. Entering class: up to 3 students.

Brooklyn College, The City University of New York State (CUNY)/State University of New York (SUNY) at Brooklyn College of Medicine

1. 8-year program (7-year option is also available).
2. Good foundation in social sciences and humanities.
3. Undergraduate summer clinical internship is offered.
4. SAT score: Most students have at least 1200.
5. Entering class: up to 25 students per year.
6. Out-of-state residents are eligible to apply.

New York University College of Arts and Sciences/New York University School of Medicine

1. 8-year program.
2. An interdisciplinary research project is required.
3. Students can major in a science or a non-science discipline.
4. Entering class: 8-10.
5. Out-of-state applicants are eligible to apply.

University of Rochester/University of Rochester School of Medicine and Dentistry

1. 8-year program.
2. Average SAT score: over 1450.

3. Entering class: up to 10.

4. Out-of-state residents are eligible to apply.

Siena College/Albany Medical College

1. 8-year program.

2. Emphasis on humanities, social service, and ethics.

3. Two summers in volunteer service (grants available for living expenses and lost summer income).

4. Most SAT scores: 1300 or greater; ACT score: 30 or better.

5. Entering class: 10-15.

6. Out-of-state residents are eligible to apply.

*Siena College/State University of New York (SUNY) Health Science Center at Syracuse College of Medicine

1. 8-year program.

2. Early Assurance Program: apply at the end of sophomore year

3. 1280 SAT score.

4. Most are science majors.

5. Average number of positions: one or two per year.

6. Limited to New York State residents.

*State University of New York(SUNY) at Buffalo/SUNY Buffalo School of Medicine

1. 8-year program.

2. Early assurance: apply as a second semester sophomore.

3. A broad education in the humanities and social sciences is also encouraged.

4. Entering class: may accept up to 25-30.

5. SUNY-Buffalo is in the New York State system of public universities: preference is given to New York State residents.

State University of New York at Stony Brook/SUNY at Stony Brook School of Medicine Health Sciences Center

1. 8-year program.

2. Apply as a high school senior.

3. Entering class: up to 5.

4. SUNY-Stony Brook is in the New York State system of public universities: preference is given to New York State residents.

*State University of New York at Stony Brook(Scholars for Medicine Program)/SUNY at Stony Brook School of Medicine Health Sciences Center

1. 8-year program.

2. Apply as a college sophomore (Scholars for Medicine Program) for early acceptance.

3. Entering class: up to 5.

4. SUNY-Stony Brook is in the New York State system of public universities: preference is given to New York State residents.

OHIO

Case Western Reserve University/Case Western Reserve University School of Medicine

1. 8-year program.

2. Students can major in a science or a non-science discipline.

3. Average SAT score: over 1400; average ACT score: over 31.

4. Entering class: 25.

5. Out-of-state residents are eligible to apply.

PENNSYLVANIA

Gannon University/Allegheny University of the Health Sciences: Medical College of Pennsylvania/Hahnemann School of Medicine

1. 8-year program.

2. SAT score: 1270 or higher.

3. Emphasis on primary care: family medicine, general pediatrics, or general internal medicine.

4. Entering class: up to 10.

5. Preference is given to residents of Northwest Pennsylvania.

Indiana University of Pennsylvania/Allegheny University of the Health Sciences: Medical College of Pennsylvania/Hahnemann School of Medicine

1. 8-year program.

2. Minimum SAT score of 1270 (no score below 550).

3. Preference is given to applicants interested in primary care (family practice, general internal medicine, or general pediatrics).

4. Entering class: up to 4.

5. Preference is given to residents of Southern Pennsylvania and the Pittsburgh area.

Muhlenberg College/Allegheny University of the Health Sciences: Medical College of Pennsylvania/Hahnemann School of Medicine

1. 8-year program.

2. College senior year internship program at Lehigh Valley Hospital.

3. Research opportunities are available.

4. Typical SAT scores: 1270 or higher.

5. Entering class: up to 6 students (if class is not filled , freshmen, sophomores, or juniors can apply for the program).

6. Preference is given to applicants from the Lehigh Valley, Eastern Pennsylvania, and New Jersey.

Rosemont College/Allegheny University of the Health Sciences: Medical College of Pennsylvania/Hahnemann School of Medicine

1. 8-year program.

2. SAT score: minimum 1300 with no score below 600.

3. Liberal arts college for women.

4. Entering class: up to 5.

5. Out-of-state female applicants are eligible to apply.

Ursinus College/Allegheny University of the Health Sciences: Medical College of Pennsylvania/Hahnemann School of Medicine

1. 8-year program.

2. Students can major in a science or a non-science discipline.

3. Minimum SAT score of 1300 (no single score less than 650).

4. Entering class: up to 6.

5. Out-of-state residents are eligible to apply.

*West Chester University/The Pennsylvania State University College of Medicine

1. 8-year program.

2. SAT standard: 1250.

3. Apply at the end of sophomore year for early acceptance.

4. Career interest in primary care medicine.

5. Biomedical research internships are available for full credit (junior year).

6. Out-of-state residents are eligible to apply.

RHODE ISLAND

Brown University/Brown University School of Medicine

The Program in Liberal Medical Education (PLME)

1. 8-year program.

2. Wide choice of majors: A.B. (Bachelor Degree) or Sc.B. Degree in the sciences or an A.B. in the Humanities, Behavioral or Social Sciences. Interdisciplinary majors also available: *e.g.* Public Policy, International Studies, Biomedical Ethics.

3. Entering class: average is 65.

4. Out-of-state residents are eligible to apply.

*Providence College, *Rhode Island College, *University of Rhode Island, *Tougaloo College (Mississippi)/Brown University School of Medicine

The Early Identification Program (EIP)

1. 8-year program.

2. Students are identified by their premedical advisor in the sophomore year of college.

3. Admitted undergraduate students participate in selected activities of the Program in Liberal Medical Education (PLME).

4. Entering class: up to 2 students may be admitted from each of the 4 schools.

5. Eligibility: Rhode Island residents or students from Tougaloo College (Mississippi).

TENNESSEE

*East Tennessee State University (ETSU) College of Arts and Sciences/East Tennessee State University James H. Quillon College of Medicine

1. 8-year program.

2. Admitted into the Premedical-Medical Program (PMMD) only after one full academic year of coursework; students apply near the end of their freshman year at East Tennessee State University (ETSU).

3. Only for "entering" ETSU students. Transfer students with more than 14 credits are not eligible.

4. ACT: 24; SAT: 1100.

5. Must obtain a B.A./B.S. (with a major or a minor in the humanities).

6. Entering class: up to 15.

7. Out-of-state applicants are eligible to apply; preference may be given to Tennessee residents.

TEXAS

Rice University/Baylor College of Medicine

1. 8-year program.

2. There are course requirements in the social sciences and humanities.

3. Entering class: up to 15.

4. Out-of-state residents are eligible to apply.

VIRGINIA

Virginia Commonwealth University/Virginia Commonwealth University Medical College of Virginia School of Medicine

Guaranteed Admissions Program

1. 8-year program.

2. Undergraduate Honors Program.

3. SAT score: minimum 1270.

4. Entering class: up to 20.

5. Out-of-state residents are eligible to apply.

*College of William and Mary, *Hampton University, *Norfolk State University, Old Dominion University/Eastern Virginia Medical School

*College of William and Mary (apply during freshman year in college).
*Hampton University (apply during freshman year in college).
*Norfolk State University (apply during freshman year in college).
 Old Dominion University (apply during senior year in high school).

1. 8-year program.

2. Acceptances: up to 25-30 positions are offered.

3. Out-of-state residents are eligible to apply.

Addresses of Combined Bachelor Degree/M.D. Programs and Early Assurance Programs

(Programs marked with an asterisk (*) require the student to apply for early acceptance as a college undergraduate [not as a high school senior].)

ALABAMA

8-Year Programs:

1. University of Alabama
   at Birmingham (UAB)
   (undergraduate school)

Office of Medical Student
Services/Admissions
ATTN: Early Medical School
Acceptance Program (EMSAP)
University of Alabama
School of Medicine, VH100
Birmingham, AL 35294-0019
(205) 934-2330
(205) 034 8724 (FAX)

2. Affiliated with the University of
   South Alabama School of Medicine

Office of Admissions
University of South Alabama
Administrative Building
Room 182
Mobile, AL 36688-0002
(800) 872-5247 or
(334) 460-6141

CALIFORNIA

7-Year Program:

Affiliated with the UCLA
School of Medicine

Student Affairs Officer
Division of Biomedical Sciences
University of California, Riverside
Riverside, CA 92521-0121
(909) 787-4333

8-Year Program:

Affiliated with the USC
School of Medicine

Office of College Academic Services
College of Letters, Arts, and Sciences
University of Southern California
Los Angeles, CA 90089-0152
(213) 740-5930

DELAWARE

8-Year Programs:

* 1. Affiliated with the Jefferson Medical
     College of Thomas Jefferson University

Admissions Office
University of Delaware
ATTN: Medical Scholars Program
116 Hullihen Hall
Newark, DE 19716-6210
(302) 831-8123
(302) 831-6905 (FAX)

2. The Delaware Institute of Medical
   Education and Research (DIMER)
   Program

Associate Dean for Admissions
Jefferson Medical College of
Thomas Jefferson University
1025 Walnut Street
Philadelphia, PA 19107
(215) 955-6983
(215) 923-6939 (FAX)

DISTRICT OF COLUMBIA

6-Year Program:

Affiliated with the Howard University
College of Medicine

Center for Preprofessional Education
PO Box 473
Administration Building
Howard University
Washington, DC 20059
(202) 238-2363

7-Year Programs:

* 1. Early Entry Medical Education
    Program (EEMEP)

Office of Admissions
Office of the Dean
ATTN: Early Entry Medical
Education Program (EEMEP)
Howard University
College of Medicine
520 W Street, NW
Washington, DC 20059
(202) 806-6270
(202) 806-7934 (FAX)

2. Affiliated with the George Washington
   University School of Medicine

Office of Admissions
George Washington University
2121 I Street, NW
Washington, DC 20052
(800) 447-3765 or
(202) 994-4654

8-Year Programs:

* 1. Affiliated with the George Washington
    University School of Medicine and Health
    Sciences

Office of Admissions
George Washington University
2121 I Street, NW
Washington, DC 20052
(800) 447-3765 or
(202) 994-4654

2. Affiliated with the Georgetown University
   School of Medicine

Early Assurance Program
Office of Undergraduate Admissions
Georgetown University
Washington, DC 20057-1002
(202) 687-3600

FLORIDA

6 or 7-Year Program:

Affiliated with the University of Miami
School of Medicine

Office of Admissions
University of Miami
PO Box 248025
Coral Gables, FL 33124
(305) 284-4323

7-Year Program:

* Junior Honors Medical Program

Office of Medical Education
ATTN: Junior Honors Medical Program
University of Florida
College of Medicine
PO Box 100213
Gainesville, FL 32610
(352) 392-3690
(352) 392-3940 (FAX)

ILLINOIS

7-Year Program:

Affiliated with the Northwestern University
School of Medicine

Office of Admissions and Financial Aid
Northwestern University
1801 Hinman Avenue
Evanston, IL 60204-3060
(847) 491-7271

8-Year Program:

Affiliated with the Finch University of
Health Sciences-Chicago Medical School

Premedical Office
Illinois Institute of Technology
10 West 32nd Street
Engineering 1 Building, Room 116
Chicago, IL 60616-3793
(312) 567-8852
(312) 567-5707 (FAX)

or

Illinois Institute of Technology
Director of Admissions
B.S./M.D. Program
10 West 33rd Street
Chicago, IL 60616
(800) 448-2329 (outside Chicago) or
(312) 567-3025

MASSACHUSETTS

7-Year Program (with 8-Year option):

Affiliated with the Boston University
School of Medicine

Assistant Director of Admissions
Boston University
121 Bay State Road
Boston, MA 02215
(617) 353-2300

8 Year Programs:

* 1. Modular Medical Integrated Curriculum
    (MMEDIC)

Boston University College of
Liberal Arts
Health Science Programs Office
Room 109
725 Commonwealth Avenue
Boston, MA 02215

* 2. Engineering/Medical Intergrated
    Curriculum (ENGMEDIC)

Boston University
Department of Biomedical Engineering
College of Engineering
ERB 401
44 Cummington Street
Boston, MA 02215-2407

3. Early Medical School Selection Program
    (EMSSP)

Early Medical School Selection Program
Boston University School of Medicine
80 East Concord Street
Room L-102
Boston, MA 02118

* 4. Affiliated with Mt. Sinai
    School of Medicine

Brandeis University
Office of Admissions
415 S. Street
Waltham, MA 02254
(617) 736-3500

* 5. Affiliated with Tufts University
    School of Medicine

Brandeis University
Office of Admissions
415 S. Street
Waltham, MA 02254
(617) 736-3500

MICHIGAN

8-Year Programs:

1. Affiliated with the University of Michigan
    Medical School

Inteflex Program
1301 Catherine Street
5101 Medical Science I Building
University of Michigan
Ann Arbor, MI 48109-0611
(313) 764-9534
(313) 936-3510 (FAX)

2. Michigan State University
    (undergraduate school)

College of Human Medicine
Office of Admissions
A-239 Life Sciences
Michigan State University
East Lansing, MI 48824
(517) 353-9620

MISSOURI

6-Year Program:

University of Missouri-Kansas City
College of Arts and Sciences or
UMKC School of Biological Sciences
(undergraduate schools)

Council on Selection
University of Missouri-Kansas City
School of Medicine
2411 Holmes
Kansas City, MO 64108-2792
(816) 235-1870
(816) 235-5277 (FAX)

NEBRASKA

7-Year Programs:

1. Affiliated with the University of Nebraska
    Medical Center, University of Nebraska
    College of Medicine

Chadron State College
Dean of the School of Science
and Mathematics
ATTN: Rural Health Opportunities
Program (RHOP)
10th and Main
Chadron, NE 69337
(308) 432-6293

2. Affiliated with the University of Nebraska Medical Center, University of Nebraska College of Medicine

Wayne State College
Division of Mathematics and Science
ATTN: Rural Health Opportunities
Program (RHOP)
Wayne, NE 68787
(402) 375-7329

3. Additional Contact:

University of Nebraska Medical Center
ATTN: Rural Health Opportunities
Program (RHOP)
600 South 42nd Street
Omaha, NE 68198-6660
(402) 559-8946

NEW JERSEY

7-Year Programs:

Affiliated with UMDNJ-
New Jersey Medical School

1. Department of Biology
   Drew University
   ATTN: UMDNJ-New Jersey Medical
   School Accelerated Program
   Madison, NJ 07940
   (201) 408-3802

2. Health Professions Committee
   Department of Biology
   Montclair State University
   Upper Montclair, NJ 07043

3. Honors Premedical Curriculum
   Engineering Science Program
   Center for Biomedical Engineering
   New Jersey Institute of Technology
   University Heights
   Newark, NJ 07102
   (201) 596-3584

4. Director of Honors
   Admissions Programs
   Stevens Institute of Technology
   Castle Point on the Hudson
   Hoboken, NJ 07030

5. Associate Vice President for
   Academic Affairs
   ATTN: UMDNJ-New Jersey Medical
   School Accelerated Program
   Richard Stockton College of New Jersey
   Pomona, NJ 08240-9988

6. The College of New Jersey
   Biology Department
   ATTN: UMDNJ-New Jersey
   Medical School Accelerated Program
   Hillwood Lakes
   CN 4700
   Trenton, NJ 08650-4700
   (609) 771-2021

7. Assistant Director of Admissions
   ATTN: UMDNJ-New Jersey Medical
   School Accelerated Program
   Boston University
   Commonwealth Avenue
   Boston, MA 02215

Office of Admissions
C653 MSB
UMDNJ-New Jersey Medical School
185 South Orange Avenue
Newark, NJ 07103-2714
(201) 982-4631

7 or 8-Year Program:

* Affiliated with UMDNJ-
Robert Wood Johnson Medical School

The Richard Stockton College
of New Jersey
ATTN: Pre-Health Professional Program
PO Box 195
Pomona, NJ 08240

8-Year Programs:

1. Affiliated with Allegheny University
   of the Health Sciences: Medical College
   of Pennsylvania/Hahnemann School of
   Medicine

Monmouth University
Office of Undergraduate Admissions
West Long Branch, NJ 07764-1898
(800) 543-9671 or
(908) 571-3456
(908) 263-5166 (FAX)

* 2. Affiliated with UMDNJ-
   Robert Wood Johnson
   Medical School

Bachelor/Medical Degree Program
Nelson Biological Laboratory
Rutgers University
PO Box 1059
Piscataway, NJ 08855-1059
(908) 445-5270

NEW YORK

6-Year Program:

Affiliated with Albany Medical College

Dean of Undergraduate Admissions
Rensselaer Polytechnic Institute
110 Eighth Street
Troy, NY 12180-3590
(518) 276-6216

7-Year Programs:

1. Affiliated with 7 New York State
   Medical Schools

Sophie Davis School of
Biomedical Education
City University of New York
Office of Admissions
Y Building, Room 205N
138th Street and Convent Avenue
New York, NY 10031
(212) 650-7708

2. Affiliated with Albany Medical College

Associate Dean of Admissions
ATTN: BS/MD Program
Union College
Schenectady, NY 12308
(888) 843-6688 or
(518) 388-6112

8-Year Programs:

1. Binghamton University
   (undergraduate school)

The Early Acceptance Program
for UMEDS
College of Medicine
State University of New York
Health Science Center at Syracuse
PO Box 1000
Binghamton, NY 13902
(607) 770-8515

2. Affiliated with SUNY-Brooklyn
   College of Medicine
   (also has a 7-year option)

Director of Admissions
Brooklyn College
1602 James Hall
Brooklyn, NY 11210
(718) 951-5044

3. Affiliated with New York University
   School of Medicine

Admissions Office
New York University
College of Arts and Science
22 Washington Square North
Room 904, Main Building
New York, NY 10003
(212) 998-4500

4. Affiliated with University of Rochester
   School of Medicine and Dentistry

Rochester Early Medical Scholars
University of Rochester

Undergraduate Admissions
Meliora Hall
Rochester, NY 14627
(716) 275-3221

5. Affiliated with Albany Medical College

Siena College
Office of Admissions
515 Loudonville Road
Loudonville, NY 12211-1462
(518) 783-2423

* 6. Affiliated with SUNY-Health Science
     Center at Syracuse College of Medicine

Siena College
Office of Admissions
515 Loudonville Road
Loudonville, NY 12211-1462
(518) 783-2423

* 7. Affiliated with SUNY-Buffalo
     School of Medicine

University at Buffalo
Medical School Admissions Office
40 Biomedical Education Building
Buffalo, NY 14214-3013
(716) 829-3467

8. Affiliated with SUNY-Stony Brook
   School of Medicine Health Sciences Center

SUNY-Stony Brook
Office of Undergraduate Admissions
118 Administration Building
Stony Brook, NY 11794-1901
(516) 632-6868
(516) 632-9027 (FAX)

* 9. Affiliated with SUNY-Stony Brook
   School of Medicine Health Sciences
   Center/Scholars for Medicine Program

SUNY-Stony Brook
Office of Undergraduate Admissions
118 Administration Building
Stony Brook, NY 11794-1901
(516) 632-6868
(516) 632-9027 (FAX)

OHIO

6 or 7-year Program:

Affiliated with Northeastern Ohio
Universities College of Medicine
(NEOUCOM)

1. Office of Undergraduate Admissions
   University of Akron
   Akron, OH 44325-20001
   (330) 972-7100

2. Undergraduate Admissions Office
   Kent State University
   PO Box 5190
   Kent, OH 44242
   (330) 672-2444

3. Admissions Office
   Youngstown State University
   1 University Plaza
   Youngstown, OH 44555-3150
   (330) 742-3150

Associate Director of Admissions
Northeastern Ohio Universities
College of Medicine
4209 State Route 44, PO Box 95
Rootstown, OH 44272-0095

(330) 325-2511
(330) 325-8372 (FAX)

8-Year Program:

Affiliated with Case Western Reserve
University School of Medicine

Assistant Director of Admissions
Office of Undergraduate Admissions
Case Western Reserve University
10900 Euclid Avenue
Cleveland, OH 44106-7055
(216) 368-4450

PENNSYLVANIA

6-Year Program:

Affiliated with Jefferson Medical College
of Thomas Jefferson University

Undergraduate Admissions Office
201 Shields Building
Box 3000
Penn State University
University Park, PA 16802
(814) 865-5471

6-Year Program (with 7-Year Option):

Affiliated with Allegheny University
of the Health Sciences: Medical College
of Pennsylvania/Hahnemann
School of Medicine

Office of Admissions
27 Memorial Drive West
Lehigh University
Bethlehem, PA 18105
(610) 758-3100

6 or 7-year Program:

Affiliated with Allegheny University of the Health Sciences: Medical College of Pennsylvania/Hahnemann School of Medicine

Office of Undergraduate Admissions
Villanova University
800 Lancaster Avenue
Villanova, PA 19085-1699
(800) 338-7927

7-Year Programs:

1. Affiliated with Allegheny University of the Health Sciences: Medical College of Pennsylvania/Hahnemann School of Medicine

Duquesne University
Pre-Health Professions' Programs
Bayer Learning Center, Ste B-101
Pittsburgh, PA 15282
(412) 396-6335
(412) 396-5587 (FAX)

2. Affiliated with Allegheny University of the Health Sciences: Medical College of Pennsylvania/Hahnemann School of Medicine

West Chester University
Office of Admissions
Emil H. Messikomer Hall
100 West Rosedale Avenue
West Chester, PA 19383
(610) 436-3411

8-Year Programs:

1. Affiliated with Allegheny University of the Health Sciences: Medical College of Pennsylvania/Hahnemann School of Medicine

Gannon University
Office of Admissions
ATTN: Hamot Medical Center
Scholars Program
109 University Square
Erie, PA 16541-0001
(800) GANNON-U or
(814) 871-7240

2. Affiliated with Allegheny University of the Health Sciences: Medical College of Pennsylvania/Hahnemann School of Medicine

Indiana University of Pennsylvania
Office of Admissions
216 Pratt Hall
Indiana, PA 15705
(412) 357-2230
(412) 357-6281 (FAX)

3. Affiliated with Allegheny University of the Health Sciences: Medical College of Pennsylvania/Hahnemann School of Medicine

Muhlenberg College
Office of Admissions
Allentown, PA 18104
(610) 821-3245

4. Affiliated with Allegheny University of the Health Sciences: Medical College of Pennsylvania/Hahnemann School of Medicine

Rosemont College
Office of Admissions
1400 Montgomery Avenue
Rosemont, PA 19010-1699
(800) 331-0708 or
(610) 526-2966
(610) 527-1041 (FAX)

5. Affiliated with Allegheny University of the Health Sciences: Medical College of Pennsylvania/Hahnemann School of Medicine

Ursinus College
Office of Admissions
PO Box 1000
Collegeville, PA 19426-1000
(610) 409-3000
(610) 489-0627 (FAX)

* 6. Affiliated with Pennsylvania State University College of Medicine

West Chester University
Office of Admissions
Emil H. Messikomer Hall
100 West Rosedale Avenue
West Chester, PA 19383
(610) 436-3411

RHODE ISLAND

8-Year Programs:

1. Affiliated with Brown University School of Medicine

The Program in Liberal Medical Education (PLME)

College Admission Office
Brown University
Box 1876
Providence, RI 02912
(401) 863-2378

* 2. Affiliated with Brown University School of Medicine

Providence College
Department of Biology
Health Professions Office
ATTN: Early Identification Program
Albertus Magnus Science Center
Providence, RI 02918-0001

or

Providence College
Office of Admissions
Harkins Hall
Providence, RI 02918
(401) 865-2535

Rhode Island College
Office of Admissions
600 Mount Pleasant Avenue
Providence, RI 02908-1991
(401) 456-8234

University of Rhode Island
Office of Undergraduate Admissions
8 Ranger Road, Suite 1
Kingston, RI 02881
(401) 874-7100

Tougaloo College
ATTN: Natural Sciences Division
500 West County Line Road
Tougaloo, MS 39174

TENNESSEE

7-Year Program:

* Affiliated with Meharry Medical College

Director, Admissions and Records
ATTN: Joint Program in Biomedical
   Sciences
Fisk University
1005 D.B. Todd, Jr. Boulevard
Nashville, TN 37208
(615) 329-8500

8-Year Program:

* Affiliated with East Tennessee
State University James H. Quillon
College of Medicine

Director, Premedical-Medical Program
Office of Medical Professions
Advisement
East Tennessee State University
PO Box 70, 592
Johnson City, TN 37614-0592
(423) 439-5602
(423) 439-6905 (FAX)

TEXAS

8-Year Program:

Rice University
(undergraduate school)

Office of Admissions
Baylor College of Medicine
One Baylor Plaza
Room 106A
Houston, TX 77030
(713) 798-4842

VIRGINIA

8-Year Programs:

1. Virginia Commonwealth University
   (undergraduate school)

Virginia Commonwealth University
Medical College of Virginia
School of Medicine
PO Box 980565
Richmond, VA 23298-0565
(804) 828-9629
(804) 828-1246 (FAX)

or

Virginia Commonwealth University
Honors Program Office
ATTN: Guaranteed Admissions Program
Richmond, VA 23284-3010
(804) 828-1803

2. Affiliated with Eastern Virginia
   Medical School

* Office of Undergraduate Admissions
  College of William and Mary
  PO Box 8795
  Williamsburg, VA 23187-8795
  (757) 221-4223

* Hampton University
  Office of Admissions
  Hampton, VA 23668
  (757) 727-5328

* Norfolk State University
  Office of Admissions
  Norfolk, VA 23504
  (757) 683-8396

  Old Dominion University
  Office of Admissions
  Norfolk, VA 23529-0050
  (757) 683-3637

Other Contact Address:

Office of Admissions
Eastern Virginia Medical School
721 Fairfax Avenue
Norfolk, VA 23507-2000
(757) 446-5812

WISCONSIN

7-Year Program:

Affiliated with University of Wisconsin
Medical School

Medical Scholars Program
University of Wisconsin
Medical School
1300 University Avenue
Room 1140 A
Madison, WI 53706
(608) 263-7561
(608) 262-2327 (FAX)

20

College Graduates, Older Applicants, and Post-Baccalaureate Programs

Older medical school applicants come from a wide variety of backgrounds and careers. Some applicants have graduated college within the last few years while others have been "out for a while" (or even longer!). The variety of backgrounds seen is impressive and includes a large number of different "first" careers. A sampling of these careers would include some of the following: educators, engineers, writers, nurses, other allied health professionals (*e.g.* physical therapists, pharmacists, nutritionists), homemakers, research scientists, businessmen/women. . . . The list really could seem endless!

Medical school admission committees realize that medicine is not practiced in a vacuum; there are a number of social, economic, and political issues that directly affect medical practice and the doctor patient relationship. What's more, sensitivity to the social, humanistic, and psychological factors that affect illness and disease are all very important in the practice of medicine. Medical school admission committees recognize that candidates with different educational or career backgrounds can bring their own unique perspectives to the practice of medicine. As a group, these non-traditional "post-baccalaureate" applicants are attractive to medical schools because of their diversified backgrounds and experiences, leadership capabilities, and interpersonal skills. Their deep motivation to become physicians is also reflected in their work ethic and personal commitment to the health care profession.

The traditional post-baccalaureate student either has no science background or has only taken a minimal number of college science/math courses. There are some colleges and universities that have formal structured programs for post-baccalaureate students. There are many other schools that allow college graduates to enroll for coursework and use the services of the premedical advisory office on an "as needed" basis.

The students who enroll in these programs have already earned their undergraduate bachelor degrees (some have Masters Degrees, Ph.D.s, or another advanced professional degree) and need to return to college to complete all/some of the premedical course requirements. Some post-baccalaureate programs are informal and extremely flexible—some students

---

register to take a few courses to finish their requirements and then apply to medical school on their own. (They are not seeking a premedical advisory recommendation letter from that school but will have their own college send a letter.)

Be aware that a number of "post-baccalaureate" applicants gain admission into medical school by "designing their own program"—they take courses at a local college or university with a well-established premedical program and proceed from there! There are numerous schools that do not even advertise that they have "formal" or "informal" programs for college graduates. Colleges and universities will usually allow students with bachelors degrees to schedule the required courses for medical school admission. The student must be aware, however, that "just taking courses" may affect your class registration and enrollment. Priority for course enrollment will go to undergraduates and other students with "matriculated status." You must carefully follow the registration rules and regulations that will allow you to become a "matriculated student" at that school. With that designation, course preregistration/registration will allow you to enroll in classes and not get "closed out of a course" because of a "non-matriculated" student status. This is very important with premedical requirements because courses are taught in sequence.

If you do proceed to apply to medical school on your own, you must still involve yourself in the following activities: 1) Health care related work—part-time/volunteer/paid—you still need to show your motivation and dedication to become a physician. 2) Maintain contact with both your original and your present undergraduate schools' premed advisory offices. As long as you are a matriculated student, you should be able to take full advantage of the premedical advisory services provided by your present school. If you take a sufficient number of credit hours at your present college, you can then later decide what school (your undergraduate institution or present one) should send your official premedical advisory letter of recommendation.

Remember that the MOST IMPORTANT FACTORS FOR ADMISSION will be the STUDENT'S QUALIFICATIONS and PERSONAL ATTRIBUTES and not the post-baccalaureate program itself; there are, however, a number of programs with established medical school admission track records. Many of these same programs are very competitive — the post-baccalaureate admission requirements will include excellent undergraduate credentials, the course of study will be extremely rigorous, and not every applicant will eventually be admitted into medical school (as with all premedical programs).

The next part of this chapter discusses the "Major Factors To Consider When Enrolling in a Post-Baccalaureate Program." That will be followed by a detailed listing of post-baccalaureate programs and will include addresses and those programs that have special admission arrangements with medical schools.

Major Factors to Consider
When Enrolling in a Post-Baccalaureate Program

POST-BACCALAUREATE ADMISSION REQUIREMENTS

Depending on the program, you may need to "formally" apply for admission. The following application materials will usually be required before an admission decision is made:

- Formal application for the program (will usually include one or more essays)
- Letters of recommendation
- SAT scores
- College transcripts

You should note that some programs may even require a formal interview for acceptance. Some programs are extremely competitive and will limit the enrollment of their post-baccalaureate class.

Many of the traditional (four-year degree, no science or minimal science background) post-baccalaureate programs also add the following qualifiers:

1. Traditional programs are not meant for those students who want to improve their GPA based on previous premedical coursework.

2. The traditional programs are not considered "remedial" and students are not permitted to retake previous premedical courses.

COURSE OFFERINGS

Traditional post-baccalaureate programs will offer the premedical core courses that are required by medical schools:

1. Inorganic Chemistry (with lab): one year
2. Introductory Biology (with lab): one year
3. Organic Chemistry (with lab): one year
4. Introductory Physics (with lab): one year

Some students will need to take college algebra/trigonometry first if they have no (or minimal) math or science background. A good foundation in algebra/trigonometry is also very important for further coursework in calculus and physics. NOTE: Calculus I and/or Calculus II (mathematics courses are recommended by many medical schools) will also be offered by these post-baccalaureate programs.

Students may also need to take additional coursework in such areas as statistics, computer science, social science, psychology, etc. to fulfill a particular medical school's admissions requirements. When enrolled in post-baccalaureate premedical coursework, the student needs to make a tentative list of the schools that he/she will probably want to apply; the prospective applicant should then check to see if there are any additional courses required for admission to these schools. You need to do this early in the process so that you can constructively plan your post-baccalaureate schedule. You do not want to start applying to the medical schools of your choice and find out that all of the requirements have not been fulfilled!

PROGRAM FLEXIBILITY

This is the strong point of most programs. If you have already completed some of the required premedical coursework, you can then finish your other requirements and perhaps take additional upper-level biology courses. Be aware that formal post-baccalaureate programs will have eligibility requirements for the minimal number of courses/credit hours to be taken at their school. These requirements may affect eligibility status for admission into the program and/or the opportunity to obtain the premedical advisory recommendation letter from that program. If a student has fulfilled all basic premedical courses except for one course, for example, he/she may not be eligible for admission into that post-baccalaureate program. It is very important to read and understand the eligibility requirements of the post-baccalaureate programs you are considering. Some programs are very "informal" and allow you to take any courses that you need or desire. They may, however, still require you to take a minimum number of credit hours at their school in order to qualify for the Premedical Advisor/Advisory Committee recommendation letter. These informal programs also understand, however, that you may seek the premedical advisory recommendation letter from your original undergraduate institution (especially if you are "only taking a few courses").

Many programs emphasize the flexibility of their curriculum: full-time or part-time status with even the opportunity to take evening classes. (Many students will still be taking the traditional premed day courses with undergraduates.) With part-time status, it is assumed that students will arrange their employment situation in order to take full advantage of their premedical education.

A very large number of students take courses full-time and are not employed. They are usually able to fulfill their premedical requirements in one to two years (with/without summer courses). Doing well in a rigorous premedical program will help prove that the student can undertake a first-year basic medical science course load in medical school.

TIME FRAME/ACADEMIC SCHEDULES

There are a variety of pathways to fulfill the premedical requirements. Choosing the "appropriate curriculum" will depend on both your academic background and the individual post-baccalaureate program. The actual time necessary to complete the premedical requirements usually takes one to two years. This may include one or more summers of coursework. Summer courses and heavy course loads are obviously the two ways to shorten the time span before you would actually apply to medical school.

Some of the most highly respected post-baccalaureate programs in this country are known for their rigorous and heavy course loads (up to three science/math courses [along with labs] per semester). Attrition rates can be high with these programs, but those who complete the requirements are considered "very competitive" for the medical school application process. Post-baccalaureate programs with extremely demanding course loads (you will be "totally immersed in the sciences") have proven repeatedly that their students can meet the challenge of a first-year basic science medical school curriculum.

In most post-baccalaureate programs, one to two years is usually the "average time" to complete your basic premedical requirements. An additional year must then be used to file applications and to interview at medical schools. Some students use this time to take upper-division biology courses (*e.g.* physiology, biochemistry, anatomy, histology, etc.) to "prime" themselves for the first year of medical school; others use the time for paid employment, to travel, or to work in a health care related activity (paid/volunteer). Some students will combine two or more of these activities before attending medical school.

PREMEDICAL ADVISORY FUNCTIONS AND POST-BACCALAUREATE STUDENTS

There will be a variety of services provided for these students and may include some/all of the following:

- Working on a course schedule
- Obtaining health-related externships or positions (paid/volunteer)
- Information on research opportunities
- Choosing where to apply
- Helping with medical school applications
- Advice on personal essays
- Composite premedical advisory letter of recommendation
- Developing interviewing skills
- Mock interviews
- MCAT reviews/test preparation
- Course tutoring
- Personal advice and counsel

TUITION/FEES/COST OF LIVING

Post-baccalaureate students should carefully review the costs of a one to three year program. They will usually be required to pay the same tuition as undergraduates and will pay for their course requirements by themselves or through a prearranged loan program (*e.g.* Stafford loan program). Some students choose to "stay close to home" in order to save money. Others make a similar decision because of family commitments and employment opportunities.

FINANCIAL AID

Grants/"out-right" scholarship aid is almost non-existent for post-baccalaureate students. Loans (*e.g.* guaranteed student loan program—Federal Stafford Loans) are available for such coursework and each post-baccalaureate program will have information on financial aid. Every school will be able to tell you the necessary steps to take for obtaining loan eligibility. Please note, for example, that it will usually be necessary for the student to be "matriculated" (registered under a formal program and not "just taking courses.")

RESIDENCY REQUIREMENTS

Be aware of the residency requirements in the state where you enroll in a post-baccalaureate program. Enrolling in such a program does not guarantee residency for purposes of medical school applications. If you enroll in an out-of-state post-baccalaureate program with the intention of applying to that state's medical schools, you must pay close attention to that state's residency requirements. Most post-baccalaureate programs require one to two years of courses—a time period sufficient to acquire state residency status (if desired).

LINKAGE WITH MEDICAL SCHOOLS

Some post-baccalaureate programs provide a number of arrangements with particular medical schools that allow admission for some of their students while they are still enrolled in their premedical studies. This allows highly qualified applicants to enter medical school right after they complete their premedical studies instead of waiting the additional year to apply.

Though each linkage arrangement is a unique agreement made between the post-baccalaureate program and that medical school, it is important to summarize the variety of factors that affect admission. (In the last part of this chapter is a list of those post-baccalaureate programs that have agreements with a variety of medical schools.) The following list of factors applies to the traditional post-baccalaureate applicant—one who did not fulfill premedical requirements as an undergraduate:

1. Students should be first time medical school applicants and currently enrolled in their post-baccalaureate program.

2. A student must complete a minimum number of required premedical courses/credit hours at that post-baccalaureate program to be considered. The appropriate minimum GPAs must also be achieved and maintained.

3. The vast majority of medical schools in such linkage programs will also require the MCAT and interviews.

4. Some linkage programs allow you to apply to only one school—if you are granted admission, you must agree to matriculate at that medical school.

5. Some programs may provide "provisional acceptances" very early (even before the student has taken one course) in the post-baccalaureate process. The student then cannot apply to any other medical school and must fulfill all of the requirements determined by the post-baccalaureate program and the medical school.

HEALTH CARE RELATED EXPERIENCE

Some post-baccalaureate programs help organize a variety of clinical experiences: examples include preceptorships with physicians, hospital externships, working in clinics, emergency room work, etc. They are usually part-time volunteer positions. Some students obtain paid part-time health care positions. If your college does not provide such opportunities, you should take the initiative and find an appropriate position. A health care related work/ volunteer experience will help show your motivation, interest, and dedication to the medical profession. Remember, however, to keep everything in the proper balance—maintaining a very good GPA along with MCAT preparation remain the top priorities!

To avoid confusion with the traditional post-baccalaureate programs (Bachelors Degree with little or no science/math background), two additional chapters in this book include other types of programs that are available to students who have graduated college and have taken their premedical requirements along with the MCAT. Many of these programs are designed as "reapplicant" programs whereas others will accept those who have fulfilled the necessary premedical requirements but need to strengthen their academic credentials. (Chapter 21, "Minority Student Opportunities," addresses reapplicant programs available for minority students; Chapter 22, "Knowing the Options If You Are Not Accepted," discusses programs [including reapplication programs] that are available to applicants who need to strengthen their academic credentials before applying to medical school.)

A list of post-baccalaureate programs with medical school linkages is presented in the last part of this chapter. There is also a second detailed list that provides colleges/universities that present themselves as offering post-baccalaureate programs. (NOTE: If you need to take your premedical requirements in your local area, make sure that the undergraduate institution has a well established premedical program and an acceptable track record of getting their applicants into medical school.)

1. <u>Colleges/Universities With Linkages to Medical Schools</u>

   (See descriptions after formal listing of programs.)

   1. Scripps College (California)
   2. Goucher College (Maryland)
   3. Tufts University (Primary Care option) (Massachusetts)
   4. Columbia University (New York)
   5. CUNY-Queens College (New York)
   6. CUNY-Hunter College (New York)
   7. New York University (New York)
   8. SUNY-Stony Brook (New York)
   9. Bryn Mawr College (Pennsylvania)
   10. Duquesne University (Pennsylvania)
   11. University of Pennsylvania (Pennsylvania)
   12. West Chester University (Pennsylvania)
   13. Bennington College (Vermont)

   The above programs are typically "traditional post-baccalaureate" programs: career change, no/minimal premedical coursework. See formal descriptions for exceptions.

2. <u>Completion of Medical School Prerequisite Courses; Upper Division Science coursework Offered</u> (These universities also offer the traditional post-baccalaureate program: career change, no/minimal premedical coursework.)

   - University of Connecticut
   - University of Miami (Florida)

3. <u>Colleges/Universities with Upper Division Coursework/Preprofessional Master Degree Programs/Reapplication Programs</u>

   (See Chapter 22, "Knowing the Options If You Are Not Accepted.")

4. <u>Colleges/Universities with Post-baccalaureate/Reapplicant Programs for Minority Students</u>

   (See Chapter 21, "Minority Student Opportunities.")

Programs with Medical School Linkages

CALIFORNIA

Scripps College
Post-Baccalaureate Premedical Program
W.M. Keck Science Center
925 North Mills Avenue
Claremont, CA 91711-5916
(909)621-8764
(909)621-8588 (FAX)

1. Typical program is 15 months (includes two summers and one academic year).

2. Part-time status is available (part-time work schedule required).

3. Linkage with the following medical schools:

    1. Temple University School of Medicine.

    2. Western University of Health Sciences, College of Osteopathic Medicine (Pomona, California).

MARYLAND

Goucher College
Post-Baccalaureate Premedical Program
1021 Dulaney Valley Road
Baltimore, MD 21204-2794
(800)697-4646 or
(410)337-6221
(410)337-6085 (FAX)

1. Typical timetable: one summer and one full academic year.

2. MCAT review sessions available.

3. Organized medical preceptorships available.

4. Linkage with the following medical schools:

    1. Allegheny University of the Health Sciences: Medical College of Pennsylvania/ Hahnemann School of Medicine.

    2. SUNY at Stony Brook School of Medicine.

    3. Temple University School of Medicine.

    4. Tulane University School of Medicine.

MASSACHUSETTS

Tufts University
ATTN: Post-Baccalaureate Premedical Program
112 Packard Avenue
Medford, MA 02155
(617)627-3562
(617) 627-3017 (FAX)

1. Limited to 40 students/year.

2. Interview granted at Tufts University School of Medicine if applicant completes the program with a minimum 3.3 GPA.

3. Additional option offered: simultaneous acceptance into the School of Medicine if committed to a career in primary care (must maintain required GPA and obtain a sufficient MCAT score).

4. Must take minimum of six science courses.

NEW YORK

1. Columbia University School of General Studies
   408 Lewisohn Hall
   2970 Broadway, Mail Code 4101
   New York, NY 10027
   (212) 854-2772

   1. Oldest and largest formal post-baccalaureate program (approximately 300 total students).

   2. Linkage with the following medical schools:

      1. Allegheny University of the Health Sciences: Medical College of Pennsylvania/ Hahnemann School of Medicine.

      2. Brown University School of Medicine.

      3. State University of New York at Stony Brook School of Medicine.

      4. Temple University School of Medicine

      5. Jefferson Medical College of Thomas Jefferson University

2. CUNY-Queens College
   Health Professions Advisory Committee
   Flushing, NY
   (718)997-3470

CUNY: City University of New York

1. Linkage with SUNY at Stony Brook School of Medicine

2. Also has traditional post-baccalaureate program

3. CUNY-Hunter College
    Pre-Professional Office
    ATTN: Post-Baccalaureate Program
    695 Park Avenue, Room 313-N
    New York, NY 10021
    (212)772-5244

    CUNY: City University of New York

    1. Linkage with SUNY at Stony Brook School of Medicine.

    2. Also has traditional post-baccalaureate program.

4. New York University
    College of Arts and Science
    Prehealth Advisement Office
    ATTN: Post-Baccalaureate Premedical Studies
    Main Building, Room 904
    100 Washington Square East
    New York, NY 10003-6688
    (212)998-8160

    1. Part-time and full-time status is available.

    2. Exposure and experiences in a health care setting are offered.

    3. Linkage with the following medical schools:

        1. SUNY at Stony Brook School of Medicine.

        2. SUNY at Syracuse College of Medicine.

        3. SUNY at Brooklyn College of Medicine.

        4. New York Medical College.

5. SUNY/Stony Brook
    School of Professional Development and Continuing Studies
    ATTN: Post-Baccalaureate Premedical Program
    Stony Brook, NY 11794-4310
    (516) 632-7050
    (516) 632-9046 (FAX)

Up to 5 places are reserved at SUNY at Stony Brook School of Medicine Health Sciences Center for Stony Brook post-baccalaureate students.

PENNSYLVANIA

1. Bryn Mawr College
    Post-Baccalaureate Premedical Program
    Canwyll House
    101 North Marion Avenue
    Bryn Mawr, PA 19010-2899
    (610) 526-7350
    (610) 526-7353 (FAX)

    1. Typical completion time: one academic year plus one or two summers.
    2. Linkage with the following medical schools:
        1. Allegheny University of the Health Sciences: Medical College of Pennsylvania/ Hahnemann School of Medicine.
        2. Brown University School of Medicine.
        3. Dartmouth Medical School.
        4. Jefferson Medical College of Thomas Jefferson University.
        5. SUNY at Brooklyn School of Medicine.
        6. SUNY at Stony Brook School of Medicine.
        7. Temple University School of Medicine.
        8. University of Rochester School of Medicine.

2. Duquesne University
    Post-Baccalaureate Premedical Program
    Suite B-101, Bayer Learning Center
    Pittsburgh, PA 15282-1502
    (412) 396-6335
    (412) 396-5587 (FAX)

    1. Post-baccalaureate programs are also open to former premedical students (with/ without a previous MCAT).
    2. Linkage eligibility: non-science degree without being enrolled as a premed student as an undergraduate.

3. Formal Introduction to Medicine Program (combines clinical experience/lectures)

4. Linkage with the following medical schools:

   1. Allegheny University of the Health Sciences: Medical College of Pennsylvania/ Hahnemann School of Medicine.

   2. Temple University School of Medicine.

   3. Lake Erie College of Osteopathic Medicine.

3. Post-Baccalaureate Prehealth Program
   College of General Studies
   University of Pennsylvania
   3440 Market Street, Suite 100
   Philadelphia, PA 19104-3335
   (215) 898-4847
   (215) 573-2053 (FAX)

   1. Two programs:

      1. Traditional: no/minimal premedical coursework.

      2. Special Science Program: refresh, complete, or improve one's science background.

   2. Day and night classes available.

   3. Volunteer clinical work available.

   4. Linkage with the following medical schools:

      1. Allegheny University of the Health Sciences: Medical College of Pennsylvania/ Hahnemann School of Medicine.

      2. Jefferson Medical College of Thomas Jefferson University.

      3. Temple University School of Medicine.

4. West Chester University
   Premedical Office
   ATTN: Post-Baccalaureate Program
   West Chester, PA 19383
   (610) 436-2978

   1. Program can be completed in one full year (including at least one summer).

   2. Linkage with the following medical schools: (see next page)

1. Allegheny University of the Health Sciences: Medical College of Pennsylvania/ Hahnemann School of Medicine.

2. Temple University School of Medicine.

VERMONT

Bennington College
Office of Admissions
Post-Baccalaureate Program
Bennington, VT 05201
(800) 833-6845
(802) 442-5401
(802) 442-6164 (FAX)

1. Two year program (four semesters).

2. Minimum of three courses per semester.

3. Linkage with Allegheny University of the Health Sciences: Medical College of Pennsylvania/ Hahnemann School of Medicine.

Regular Post-Baccalaureate Programs

ARIZONA

Post-Baccalaureate Premedical Program
Pre-Health Professions Office
McClintock Hall, Room 110B
Tempe, AZ 85287-3102
(602)965-2365
(602)965-1093 (FAX)

CALIFORNIA

1. California State University
   Dominguez Hills
   School of Science, Mathematics, and
   Technology
   Post-Baccalaureate Premedical Program
   1000 East Victoria Street
   Carson, CA 90747
   (310)243-3376

2. California State University, Fullerton
   Health Professions Committee
   Post-Baccalaureate Program
   PO Box 6848
   Fullerton, CA 92834-3980

- Assistance is available for obtaining appropriate research and/or clinical experience.

3. California State University, Hayward
   Medical Sciences Advising Committee
   Post-Baccalaureate Program
   School of Science/Office of the Dean
   25800 Carlos Bee Boulevard
   Hayward, CA 94542
   (510)885-3441
   (510)885-2035 (FAX)

4. Loyola Marymount University
   Health Professions Qualifications Committee
   Post-Baccalaureate Premedical Program
   Loyola Boulevard at West 80th Street
   Los Angeles, CA 90045-2699
   (310)338-5954

   - Students register as non-degree students on a space-available basis.

5. Mills College
   Office of Graduate Studies
   ATTN: Post-Baccalaureate Premedical Program
   5000 MacArthur Boulevard
   Oakland, CA 94613
   (510)430-3309

   - The average time of completion is one or two years.

CONNECTICUT

Post-Baccalaureate Program
University of Connecticut Health Center
School of Medicine
263 Farmington Avenue

Farmington, CT 06030-1905
Two programs are offered:
- Traditional: career change or no/minimal premedical courses.
- Students have completed medical school prerequisites: upper division science course work is offered.

DISTRICT OF COLUMBIA

Post-Baccalaureate Premedical Program
Premedical Advisory Committee
Georgetown University
37th and O Streets, NW
Washington, DC 20057
(202)687-5913

FLORIDA

University of Miami
College of Arts and Sciences
Premedical Post-Baccalaureate Program
Committee on Premedical Studies
PO Box 248004
Coral Gables, FL 33124
(305)284-5176

Two programs are offered:
- Program A: traditional post-baccalaureate program (average 1.5–2 years for completion).
- Program B: upper division courses for students who have fulfilled premedical requirements (average: one year).
- Clinical and research opportunities are available at the School of Medicine.

GEORGIA

1. Armstrong Atlantic State University
   Department of Chemistry and Physics
   Post-Baccalaureate Premedical Program
   11935 Abercon Street
   Savannah, GA 31419 1997
   (912)927-5304
   (912)921-5876 (FAX)

   • One or two year course curriculums are offered (average completion time).
   • Hospital externships available.

2. Postbaccalaureate Premedical Program for Women
   Office of Graduate Studies
   Agnes Scott College
   141 East College Avenue
   Decatur, GA 30030-3797
   (404)638-6252

INDIANA

Post-Baccalaureate Program
Department of Biology
Indiana University—Purdue University at Indianapolis
723 West Michigan Street
Indianapolis, IN 46202-5132

Two programs are offered:
• Traditional: no/minimal science background.
• Students who have completed premedical-courses: a Preprofessional Non-Thesis Master of Science Degree is offered.

ILLINOIS

1. Rosary College
   Department of Natural Sciences
   Post-Baccalaureate Premedical Program
   7900 West Division Street
   River Forest, IL 60305
   (708)366-2490

2. Loyola University Chicago
   Mundelein College
   Post-Baccalaureate Prehealth Professions Program
   Lake Shore Campus
   6525 North Sheridan Road
   Chicago, IL 60626-5385
   (312)508-6054

   • Students usually attend classes on a part-time basis. Admission for full-time status is also available.

IOWA

1. Drake University
   Department of Biology
   Post-Baccalaureate Premedical Program
   Olin Hall
   Des Moines, IA 50311
   (515)271-3925
   (515)271-3702 (FAX)

   • Suggested completion time: two semesters plus one summer.

2. Iowa State University
   Student Academic Services
   Post-Baccalaureate Premedical Program
   102 Carrie Chapman Catt Hall
   Ames, IA 50011-1302
   (515)294-4831
   (515)294-7446 (FAX)

   • Students apply as senior premedical students in the College of Liberal Arts and Sciences.

KENTUCKY

Brescia College
Admissions Office
ATTN: Post-Baccalaureate Premedical Program
717 Frederica Street
Owensboro, KY 42301-3023
(800)264-1234
(502)686 4241
(502)686-4266 (FAX)

MARYLAND

Towson State University
Biology Department
Post-Baccalaureate Premedical Program
Towson, MD 21252
(410)830-3042

• Suggested completion time for a full-time student: 12–14 months.

MASSACHUSETTS

1. Post-Baccalaureate Premedical Program
   Division of Natural Sciences
   Assumption College
   500 Salisbury Street
   PO Box 15005
   Worchester, MA 01615-0005
   (508)767-7295

2. Boston University
   College of Arts and Sciences
   Office of the Dean
   Post-Baccalaureate Premedical Program
   725 Commonwealth Avenue
   Boston, MA 02215
   (617)353-4866

3. Brandeis University
   Post-Baccalaureate Premedical Program
   PO Box 9110
   Waltham, MA 02254-9110
   (617)736-3460

4. Harvard University Extension School
   Health Careers Program
   51 Brattle Street
   Cambridge, MA 02138-3722
   (617)495-2926

   • Most students require two years to complete the required courses.

5. Mount Holyoke College
   The Frances Perkins Program
   South Hadley, MA 01075-1435
   (413)538-2077
   (413)538-3013 (FAX)

   • College graduates may pursue premedical studies through the above program.

6. Simmons College
   Dorothea Lynde Dix Scholars Program
   ATTN: Post-Baccalaureate
   Premedical Program
   300 The Fenway
   Boston, MA 02115
   (617)521-2502
   (617)521-3199 (FAX)

   • One can apply as a special student or pursue a second bachelors degree.
   • Program is also open to male college graduates.

7. Wellesley College
   Health Professions Advisory Committee
   Post-Baccalaureate Premedical Program
   Science Center
   106 Central Street
   Wellesley, MA 02181-8289
   (617)283-3150

MONTANA

The University of Montana
Post-Baccalaureate Premedical
Sciences Program
Division of Biological Sciences
Missoula, MT 59812-1002
(406)243-5122
(406)243-4184 (FAX)

• Average duration: two years.
• MCAT review assistance is available.
• Volunteer preceptorship with a local physician is available.

NEW JERSEY

1. Post-Baccalaureate Programs in the
   Health Sciences
   Premedical Advisory Department
   Ramapo College
   505 Ramapo Valley Road
   Mahwah, NJ 07430-1680
   (201)529-7727
   (201)529-7637 (FAX)

   • Typical program: one summer and one full academic year.
   • Health sciences internship (optional) is available.

2. Post-Baccalaureate Premedical Program
   Rutgers University
   Health Professions Advisory Center
   A119 Nelson Biology Laboratories
   Busch Campus
   PO Box 1059
   Piscataway, NJ 08855-1059
   (908)445-5667

NEW YORK

1. Barnard College
   Columbia University
   Office of the Dean of Studies
   Premedical Post-baccaluareate Program
   3009 Broadway
   New York, NY 10027-6598
   (212)854-2024
   (212)854-7491 (FAX)

   • To be eligible, you must be a female college graduate of a Seven Sister College: Bryn Mawr, Mt. Holyoke, Harvard–Radcliffe, Smith College, Vassar, Wellesley, or Barnard College.

2. The City University of New York—
   Queens College
   Health Professions Advisory Committee
   ATTN: Post-Baccalaureate
   Preprofessional Studies
   65-30 Kissena Boulevard
   Flushing, NY 11367-0904
   (718)997-3470

3. Long Island University
   Director, Division of Science
   Post-Baccalaureate Premedical Program
   Brooklyn, NY 11201
   (718)488-1209

4. Manhattanville College
   Office of Adult and Special Programs
   Post-Baccalaureate Premedical Program
   2900 Purchase Street
   Purchase, NY 10577
   (914)694-3425
   (914)694-3488 (FAX)

   • Suggested time of completion: two full
   academic years.

NORTH CAROLINA

University of North Carolina at Greensboro
Department of Biology
Premedical Advisory Committee
312 Eberhart Building
Greensboro, NC 27412-5001
(910)334-5391
(910)334-5839 (FAX)
• Students can complete requirements in one
  full year: two summers and one academic year.

OHIO

Post-Baccalaureate Programs/MedPath Office
The Ohio State University
College of Medicine
1178 Graves Hall
333 West 10th Avenue
Columbus, OH 43210-1239
(614)292-3161
(614)688-4041 (FAX)

• Traditional program: career change option
  (Students who have not taken or completed
  the premedical requirements.).
• Academic Enrichment Program is available
  for those who have completed premedical
  coursework.
• Physician mentoring program offered.
• Community service projects offered.
• Summer science MCAT review.
• One to three year programs.

PENNSYLVANIA

1. Albright College
   Health Sciences Advisory Committee
   ATTN: Post-Baccalaureate Program
   PO Box 15234
   Reading, PA 19612-5234
   (610)921-2381

   • Health-care externship is offered.
   • MCAT preparation course.

2. Post-Baccalaureate Premedical Program
Eberly College of Science
The Pennsylvania State University
213 Whitmore Laboratory
University Park, PA 16802-6101
(814) 863-0284 or
(814) 865-7620
(814) 863-1003 (FAX)

• Program is usually 15 months and is for students who do not have a science background.
• Flexible scheduling is available.
• There is access to tutoring, MCAT prep courses, and health-related volunteer programs.

TENNESSEE

Lipscomb University
Admissions Office
ATTN: Postbaccalaureate Pre-Medical Program
3901 Granny White Pike
Nashville, TN 37204-3951
(800) 333-4358 ext. 1776

TEXAS

1. Lamar University
Post-Baccalaureate Premedical Program
Department of Chemistry
PO Box 10022
Beaumont, TX 77710
(409) 880-8267
(409) 880-8270 (FAX)

• Research projects with faculty members are available.

2. The University of Texas at Arlington
Office of the Dean/College of Science
Post-Baccalaureate Premedical Program
PO Box 19047
Arlington, TX 76019-0047
(817) 272-3491
(817) 272-3511 (FAX)

• Typical program involves 1 1/2 academic years and summer courses.

VIRGINIA

Old Dominion University
College of Sciences
Department of Biological Sciences
Premedical Post-Baccalaureate Program
Norfolk, VA 23529-0266
(757) 683-3595
(757) 683-5283 (FAX)

• Offers some courses that are taught in conjunction with the Eastern Virginia Medical School.

WASHINGTON

Seattle University
Premedical Advisory Committee
Post-Baccalaureate Program
Broadway and Madison
900 Broadway
Seattle, WA 98122-4340
(206) 296-5486
(206) 296-5634 (FAX)

• Most post-baccalaureate students volunteer in health-related science programs.

21
Minority Student Opportunities

There are a variety of opportunities available to minority group students who are under-represented in the practice of medicine. (These groups include Native Americans, African-Americans, mainland Puerto Ricans, and Mexican Americans. Students from socio-economically disadvantaged backgrounds also have access to a number of these programs.) As with all medical school applicants, the motivation and commitment to become a physician and the opportunity to be academically prepared are all major factors relating to ultimate success. There are numerous programs available for minority group students from the high school years through medical school. Before one looks at some of these programs, it is important to consider the following list of factors:

1. Some medical schools sponsor outreach programs to high school students. If your college guidance office does not have information on such programs, you should contact the medical school(s) in your city or state.

2. Minority students can complete a questionnaire when they take the MCAT. The Medical Minority Applicant Registry (Med-MAR) is a program sponsored by the Association of American Medical Colleges (AAMC). If the applicant participates, his/her biographical information and MCAT scores can be sent to all United States medical schools.

3. There are a variety of enrichment programs—descriptions of many of them can be found in the next section of this chapter. Many of these programs offer preparation for the MCAT and techniques for test-taking.

4. Minority students who are reapplying to medical school should look at the last section of this chapter. There is a general description of these opportunities along with a list of some of these programs.

5. Medical schools usually have either a Minority Affairs Office or a contact person in one of the other administrative offices (*e.g.* Dean of Student Affairs, Special Programs Office, Multicultural Affairs Office, etc.). When applying to medical school, it is important to contact these offices about their programs.

6. The AAMC publishes *Minority Student Opportunities in United States Medical Schools,*

13th edition, 1996. Association of American Medical Colleges, Department 66, Washington, DC 20055; Telephone (202)828-0416.

For additional information, minority students can also contact the AAMC at the following address:

Minority Student Information Clearinghouse
Division of Community and Minority Programs
Association of American Medical Colleges
2450 N Street, NW
Washington, DC 20037-1126

7. You can also receive information on publications for minority students by contacting the following address: Office of Statewide Health Planning and Development, Health Professions Career Opportunity Programs, 1600 Ninth Street, Room 441, Sacramento, California 95814.

8. You can obtain information on financial aid by reading Chapter 24 of this book, ("Financing Your Medical School Education"). Information on minority student application and acceptance rates can be found in Chapter 17, "Statistics for Premedical Students" (Table 6).

9. Some medical schools have summer enrichment programs for medical students who are beginning their first year studies. You should inquire about the availability of these programs at the schools where you are applying.

10. The next section has a list of summer programs (with short descriptions) in the following areas: Enrichment Programs, MCAT Preparation, and Medical/Biomedical Research. Details of these programs may change (*e.g.* funding, application deadline dates, housing arrangements, stipends, etc.) so it is important for the student to contact them directly; because application deadlines vary, you should send for information early in the academic year.

Summer College Enrichment Programs

Minority Medical Education Program (MMEP)
Association of American Medical Colleges
Division of Community and Minority Programs
2450 N. Street, NW
Washington, DC 20037-1127
(202) 828-0401
(202) 828-1125 (FAX)

- MMEP is sponsored by the Robert Wood Johnson Foundation.

- Some program highlights include:
  1. Academic enrichment (*e.g.* biology, math, etc.).
  2. MCAT preparation and review.
  3. Clinical/research mentorship.
  4. Review and counseling regarding the medical school application process.

- One centralized application is processed by the AAMC; participating institutions include the following:

  1. Alabama
  2. Baylor/Rice University
  3. Case Western Reserve
  4. Chicago Consortium Sites: Northwestern, Loyola, University of Chicago, and Rush University
  5. Vanderbilt/Fisk University
  6. University of Virginia
  7. University of Washington
  8. Yale University

- Students must have completed one year of college (NOTE: Postbaccalaureate students are eligible.).

- Information about the participating school programs will be sent to you by MMEP/AAMC at the previously listed address.

CALIFORNIA

Pre-Medical Enrichment Program
Office of Student Support Services
13-154 CHS
UCLA School of Medicine
Los Angeles, CA 90095-1720
(310) 825-3575

- Program one: includes problem solving and clinical preceptorships (minimum one year of college chemistry).

- Program two: similar to first program plus MCAT preparation. Students must have the following minimum requirements: one year of college biology, chemistry, math, and one semester of physics.

HePP Program
Office of Minority Affairs
University of Southern California
School of Medicine
1333 San Pablo St., MCH 51-C
Los Angeles, CA 90033
(213) 342-1050

- HePP Program: Health Professional Preparation.

- A variety of programs are available including preparation for college chemistry, biology, math, calculus, organic chemistry and the MCAT.

- There is also a program for high school students.

CONNECTICUT

College Enrichment Program
University of Connecticut Health Center
Office of Minority Student Affairs
Farmington, CT 06030-3920
(860) 679-3483

- Courses in biology, organic chemistry, biochemistry, physics, and calculus are offered.

- Lectures/labs/ directed study.

- College freshmen and sophomores.

Office of Minority Student Affairs
University of Connecticut
Health Center
Medical/Dental Preparatory Program
Farmington, CT 06030-3920
(860) 679-3483

- Basic medical science lectures.
- MCAT preparation.
- College junior/senior or recent preprofessional program graduate.

DISTRICT OF COLUMBIA

Summer Health Careers
Advanced Enrichment Program
Center for Preprofessional Education
Howard University
Box 473, Administrative Building
Washington, DC 20059
(202) 806-7231

- Basic science course review.
- MCAT preparation.
- Eligibility: junior/senior, completion of basic science requirements.

LOUISIANA

Summer Reinforcement and Enrichment
  Program (SREP)
Office of MEDREP and Student Services
Tulane University Medical Center
1430 Tulane Ave. SL40
New Orleans, LA 70112
(504) 588-5327

- MEDREP: Medical Education Reinforcement and Enrichment Program
- Clinical research and medical preceptorships.
- Basic science and MCAT review sessions and interviewing skills.
- At least two years of college science. Preference is given to those who have

completed their junior year of college or recent postbaccalaureate students preparing for admission to a health professions training program.

MASSACHUSETTS

Program Director
Summer Enrichment Program
Office of Outreach Programs
University of Massachusetts
Medical Center
55 Lake Ave. N.
Worcester, MA 01655
(508) 856-5541
(508) 856-4888 (FAX)

- Eligibility: minimum thirty hours college credit.
- Organic chemistry desired.
- Focus on physics and physiology.
- MCAT preparatory sessions.
- Massachusetts state resident.

MINNESOTA

Multicultural Institute
Academic Health Center
University of Minnesota
1-125 Moos Tower
515 Delaware Street SE
Minneapolis, MN 55455
(612) 624-9400

- Students must be entering college or continuing college studies in the fall.
- Separate programs in general chemistry, physics, biology, and organic chemistry.

NORTH CAROLINA

Science Enrichment Preparation Program
North Carolina Health Careers Access
  Program
University of North Carolina at Chapel Hill
CB# 8010-301 Pittsboro Street, Suite 351
Chapel Hill, NC 27599-8010
(919)966-2264
(919)966-6109 (FAX)

- Preparation in physics, organic chemistry, human physiology, quantitative skills/ biostatistics.
- Standardized test-taking skills.
- Admission skills seminar and workshop.

College Phase Summer Program
Office of Minority Affairs
Wake Forest/Bowman Gray School of
  Medicine
Medical Center Boulevard
Winston - Salem, NC 27157-1037
(919) 716-4201

- College science and mathematics preparation.
- Entering freshman or sophomore year.

Upper Level Premedical Institute
Office of Minority Affairs
Wake Forest/Bowman Gray School of
  Medicine
Medical Center Boulevard
Winston - Salem, NC 27157-1037
(919) 716-4201

- Basic premedical sciences course review.
- MCAT preparation.
- Mock admission interviews.
- Entering junior/senior year in college.

OHIO

HCEM Program
Minority Programs Office
Case Western Reserve University
School of Medicine
10900 Euclid Avenue
Cleveland, OH 44106-4920
(216) 368-1914

- HCEM: Health Careers Enhancement Program for Minorities.
- Lectures/laboratory experience.
- Medical school application counseling.
- MCAT test-taking drills.

Summer Scholars Program
Premedical Education Office
Ohio University College of Osteopathic
  Medicine
Center of Excellence
030 Grosvenor Hall
Athens, OH 45701
(614) 593-0892

- Principles of basic medical sciences/ research and demonstrative projects/principles of osteopathic medicine/study strategies.
- Minimum one year each of undergraduate college biology and chemistry.

- Preference to rising seniors, and postbaccalaureate students.

Summer Premedical Enrichment Program
University of Cincinnati
College of Medicine
Office of Student Affairs and Admissions
231 Bethesda Ave.
Cincinnati, OH 45267-0552

- Physician mentorships.
- Introduction to basic medical science classes.
- Mock interview for medical school.
- Undergraduate level: juniors and seniors (completion of college biology and general chemistry).

OKLAHOMA

Headlands Indian Health Careers Summer
    Program
University of Oklahoma Health Sciences
    Center
BSEB, Room 200
PO Box 26901
Oklahoma City, OK 73126-9968
(405) 271-2250

- Mini-block courses in basic premedical sciences and calculus.
- American Indian students who are high school seniors or college freshmen.

PENNSYLVANIA

Summer Premedical Academic Enrichment
    Program
Office of Student Affairs/Minority Programs
University of Pittsburgh
School of Medicine
M-247 Scaife Hall
Pittsburgh, PA 15261
(412) 648-8987
(412) 648-1236 (FAX)

- For entering college freshmen: goal is to strengthen academic skills; interaction with medical students and doctors.
- College junior and senior students: skill training for standardized tests and interviews. Exposure to a hospital environment.

TEXAS

Bridge to Medicine Summer Program
Office of Student Affairs and Admissions
Texas A&M University Health Center
College of Medicine
106 Reynolds Medical Building
College Station, TX 77843-1114
(409) 862-4065

- Basic sciences and MCAT prep course.
- Clinical preceptorships.
- Mock interviews.
- Eligibility: minimum sixty credit hours of college coursework, including eight hours each of biology/organic chemistry, general physics and three hours each in math and English.

Summer MCAT Preparation Course

Summer MCAT Preparation Program
Center for Educational Achievement
Charles R. Drew University
School of Medicine and Science
1621 East 120th St.
Los Angeles, CA 90059
(213) 563-4926
(213) 563-1953 (FAX)

- Preparation for every section of the MCAT.
- Mock exams.
- Academic counseling.

Medical/Biomedical Research

CONNECTICUT

Summer Research Fellowship Program
University of Connecticut Health Center
Office of Minority Student Affairs
Farmington, CT 60303-3920
(860) 679-3483

- Research experience.
- Exposure to clinical medicine.
- College sophomores, juniors, or seniors.
- Completion of some college courses in biology and chemistry (preferably through organic chemistry).

MARYLAND

NINDS Summer Program in the Neurosciences
    Office
National Institute of Health
Building 31, Room 8A19
Bethesda, MD 20892
(301) 496-5322

NINDS: National Institute of Neurological Disorders and Stroke

1. Training in neuroscience research.
2. Lectures and seminars.
3. High school (at least 16 years of age), undergraduate, graduate, and medical students are eligible to apply.

MASSACHUSETTS

Summer Honors Undergraduate Research
  Program
Programs for Minority Science Students
Harvard Medical School
Division of Medical Science
260 Longwood Avenue
Boston, MA 02115
(800) 367-9019 or
(617) 432-4980

- Students should be entering junior or
  senior year in college.

- Previous research experience.

- Strong interest in a research career.

Summer Research Program for Undergraduate
  Students
Tufts University
Sackler School of Graduate
Biomedical Sciences
136 Harrison Avenue
Boston, MA 02111
(617) 636-6767

- Laboratory research.

- Workshops on medical/graduate school
  admission.

Research Fellowship Program
Office of Student Services
University of Massachusetts Medical Center
55 Lake Avenue North
Worcester, MA 01655-0132
(508) 856-2444 or
(508) 856-5033
(508) 856-4888 (FAX)

- Research areas: Cardiovascular, pulmonary,
  hematologic diseases and sleep disorders.

- Undergraduate, graduate, and health professional school students.

NEW YORK

Cornell University Medical College
The Travelers Summer Research Fellowship
  Program for Premedical Minority Students
1300 York Avenue, Room D-119
New York, NY 10021
(212) 746-1057

- Research project.

- Lecture series, seminars, and hospital
  rounds.

- Entering senior year of college.

NHLBI Program
Office of Ethnic and Multicultural Affairs
University of Rochester School of Medicine
  and Dentistry
Box 601
Rochester, NY 14642
(716) 275-2928

- NHLBI: National Heart, Lung, and Blood
  Institute.

- Undergraduates interested in biomedical
  research careers.

Office of Ethnic and Multicultural Affairs
Summer Research Fellowship Program
University of Rochester School of Medicine
    and Dentistry
601 Elmwood Ave., Box 601
Rochester, NY 14642
(716) 275-2928

- Includes basic medical science disciplines.
- Research experience in association with a faculty member.
- Weekly seminars and workshops.
- At least two years of college.

OHIO

Pathways to Health Careers
EHCO Program
University of Cincinnati
College of Medicine
231 Bethesda Avenue
PO Box 670552
Cincinnati, OH 45267-0552
(513) 558-7212
(513) 558-1165 (FAX)

- EHCO: Environmental Health Career Opportunities.
- Biomedical research related to environmental health.
- Lectures, journal clubs, discussion of ethical issues in biomedical research.

MARC/MBRS Scholars Program
University of Cincinnati
College of Medicine
231 Bethesda Avenue
PO Box 670552
Cincinnati, OH 45267-0552
(513) 558-7212
(513) 558-1165 (FAX)

- MARC/MBRS Scholars: Minority Access to Research Careers/Minority Biomedical Research Support Scholars.
- In-depth exposure to biomedical research.
- Clinical and research conferences.
- Career counseling.
- Eligibility: (1) Enrolled in a college or university which receives MARC/MBRS funding. (2) 2 years of college with at least one year of science courses. (3) Completion of at least one year of research experience.

Pathways to Health Careers
REACH Program
University of Cincinnati
College of Medicine
231 Bethesda Avenue
PO Box 670552
Cincinnati, OH 45267-0552
(513) 558-7212
(513) 558-1165 (FAX)

- REACH: Research, Education, and Achievement for Careers in Health.
- Biomedical research related to cardiovascular, hematological health, and pulmonary sciences.
- Lectures, journal club, discussion of ethical issues in biomedical research.

TEXAS

Honors Premedical Academy
Division of School Based Programs
Baylor College of Medicine
1709 Dryden, Suite 545
Houston, TX 77030
(800) 798-8244 or
(713) 798-8200

- Laboratory/clinical research.

- MCAT preparation.

- Minimum one year of college.

- Post-baccalaureate students are also eligible.

Post-Baccalaureate Reapplicant Programs

Academic Enrichment Programs

These programs help students improve their academic and personal credentials and make them more competitive in the application process. Listed below are examples of some of the program attributes and strengths that a student should look for when considering such a course of study (The completion of all premedical coursework is usually a prerequisite in the reapplication programs.):

1. Strategies to use when reapplying.

2. Formal MCAT reviews and preparation.

3. Mock interviews.

4. Opportunities to improve basic premedical science course grades.

5. Upper division science coursework (especially those in the biological sciences and some courses which may be taken during the first year in medical school).

6. Programs that include regular academic year schedules (with/without summer course schedules).

7. Summer programs that focus on coursework and overall personal improvement (*e.g.* time management, test-taking, and problem-solving skills) for both the upcoming application cycle and for medical school.

8. Financial aid (loans, grants, tuition waivers, stipends).

9. Research projects and/or preceptorships (hospitals, clinics/doctors' offices).

10. Some programs offer provisional acceptance into medical school.

CALIFORNIA

Post-Baccalaureate Program
Office of Minority Affairs
University of California, Davis
School of Medicine
Davis, CA 95616
(916)752-1852

- Must be a California resident.
- Summer and two academic quarters.

Post-Baccalaureate Program
Student Outreach Services
University of California, San Diego
School of Medicine
Date Building, Room 107
9500 Gillman Drive
La Jolla, CA 92093-0655
(619) 534-4170

- Must be a California resident.
- Summer and one full academic year.

CONNECTICUT

Post-Baccalaureate Program
University of Connecticut Health Center
School of Medicine
263 Farmington Avenue
Farmington, CT 06030-1905

- Programs for students who either have or have not completed premedical science prerequisites.
- Two summers and one academic year.

ILLINOIS

MEDPREP
Southern Illinois University
School of Medicine
Wheeler Hall
Carbondale, IL 62901-4323
(618) 536-6671

- MEDPREP: Medical Education Preparatory Program
- Eighteen months to two years.
- Students need not have taken the MCAT or applied to medical school.

MICHIGAN

ATTN: Postbaccalaureate Program/
Prematriculation Programs
College of Human Medicine
Michigan State University
A-254 Life Sciences Building
East Lansing, MI 44824-1317
(517) 355-2404

- Must have applied previously to the College of Human Medicine (Michigan State University).
- Possible to receive a conditional acceptance into medical school.

Office of Student and Minority Affairs
University of Michigan Medical School
1301 Catherine Road
5109 C Medical Science I Building
Ann Arbor, MI 48109-0611
(313) 764-8185

- Preference given to Michigan residents.
- Approximately one full year.
- Possible to receive a conditional acceptance into medical school.

NEW YORK

Post-Baccalaureate Program
State University of New York at Buffalo
School of Medicine and Biomedical Science
3435 Main Street
40 CFS Building
Buffalo, NY 14214
(716) 829-2811

Participating Medical Schools
- Mt. Sinai Medical College
- New York Medical College
- SUNY at Buffalo/Brooklyn/Stony Brook/ Syracuse
- University of Rochester
- Student must have been interviewed and denied admission into one of the above participating medical schools.

NORTH CAROLINA

Office of Minority Affairs
Bowman Gray School of Medicine
Medical Center Boulevard
Winston-Salem, NC 27157-1037
(910) 716-4201

- Possible to receive a conditional acceptance into medical school.

22

Knowing the Options
If You Are Not Accepted

If you are not admitted into medical school, by all means, do not feel alone. The application process has become so overly competitive that nearly two out of every three applicants will not be admitted. Looking at the application trends, the numbers look like they will remain that way at least into the near future. What's more, some class sizes are being cut back and there are "no big plans" (as in the 1960s - 1970s) to start financing brand new medical schools.

Unfortunately, every year thousands of applicants remain baffled by the mystique of admission committees' decisions and ask the same heart-wrenching questions: "Why wasn't I chosen?" "What does it REALLY take to get admitted?" "I thought I was qualified?!" For some students, the areas of weakness may be obvious: low or below average GPAs and/or MCAT scores. Other students, especially those with acceptable/very good quantitative criteria (GPAs and MCATs), may have to search a little deeper for factors affecting their admission. For other students, the process may become even more frustrating; they may have received numerous interviews and may have been placed on waiting lists but the end result was the same—no acceptance letter.

With the admissions process so overly competitive, premedical students have to be emotionally and mentally prepared for the possibility of medical school rejection. Realizing that this happens to nearly two out of three applicants should motivate students to carefully consider alternative plans for the following academic year(s). Remember, there are different OPTIONS to consider, but before you organize any contingency plans, you must first do a careful self-examination of the factor(s) that may have contributed to your rejection letters. You really need to be "open with yourself": only through a critical self-evaluation can you hope to learn about yourself and turn weaknesses into strengths. To help you with this insight, it would benefit you to talk to those who may have played a role in your application process: your premed advisor, the premed advisory committee at school, career and guidance counselors, and those who wrote your letters of recommendation. Furthermore, you could write or set up (only if practical, especially geographically) an appointment with medical school admission office personnel, committee members, or interviewers at the school where you were rejected, received interviews, and/or were "wait listed." Some medical schools may respond with the SPECIFICS of why you were not accepted (if they do, you should ask them what you should do to enhance your chances of admission to THAT school) while others respond with a true but GENERIC answer: "Competition for the first-year medical class was extremely competitive this year, and the applicants outnumbered the available positions."

There are a number of factors to consider when analyzing the weaknesses that may have played a role in not being accepted. Although the list may not be all-inclusive, it will help the applicant in his/her very first critical step of self-evaluation.

Factors to Consider When Reassessing Your Medical School Application

1. Low GPA (A very common factor; you need to look at both the cumulative GPA and the science GPA).

2. Low MCAT scores.

3. Low GPA and low MCAT scores.

4. Average to excellent GPA with lower MCAT scores/or good MCAT scores but lower GPA that does not reflect your standardized scores.

5. Missing certain deadlines (e.g. primary application, secondary application, submission of MCAT scores, etc.).

6. Poor or inadequate letters of recommendation.

7. "Typos," misspellings, bad grammar, and syntax in the application.

8. Personal essay.

9. Applied to only the top medical schools.

10. Applied to relatively few schools.

11. Did not select an adequate combination (private/state) of medical schools.

12. Grade "slippage."

13. Poor or less than optimal interview(s).

14. Number of times one has applied to medical school. Some reapply two, three, or four times and do not get admitted.

15. Personal qualities or characteristics that may have become evident/"misunderstood" in one part of the application process (e.g. during an interview or your personal essay).

16. Lack of evidence for true motivation or interest in practicing medicine.

17. Lack of extracurricular or volunteer activities.

18. No evidence of leadership skills.

19. Insufficient research activities (provided your initial intent was to be a research-oriented physician).

20. Too many course withdrawals or "retakes."

21. Pass/fail curriculum; too many pass/fail grades.

22. A basic science course(s) taken pass/fail.

23. Lack of exposure to hospital/clinical medicine.

For some students, one problem area may have been CRITICAL in the application process; for others, a variety of factors may have contributed to the unsuccessful applications. No matter what the factors are, rejected candidates need to take the INITIATIVE; YOU need to NURTURE YOUR OWN SUCCESS. There are ways to open those medical school admission doors, but you need to investigate the options that WILL WORK BEST FOR YOU. You have to take a positive outlook, be confident, and create a "win/win situation." What this means is the choices that you make over the next one to three (or even four) years should put you in a situation where you can achieve both personal growth and educational maturity ("be really prepared" for medical school) and also receive that much coveted letter of acceptance.

It is during this time that you will probably discover your true motivations for becoming a physician. If you are "true to yourself" in this self-awareness process, you will have the insight to make the right decision about your future. Economic gain, seeking professional prestige, or satisfying another family member's wish for you to become a doctor are NOT the RIGHT REASONS to seek a medical degree. There are other professions and careers that could make you both wealthier and more prominent if you seek those attributes.

If there is NO OTHER CHOICE FOR YOU but to become a PHYSICIAN. . . . Then proceed and never look back! That may even mean attending a foreign medical school, but remember that there are many good and successful American physicians who sought their medical education elsewhere because they were never accepted into a U.S. medical school.

Keeping all of this in mind, there are a number of options to consider if you are not accepted into medical school (The options are in no particular order and are subject to an individual's own choices):

1. Reapply during the next academic school year.

2. Enroll in a masters degree or Ph.D. program, and then reapply to medical school. Medical schools will usually want you to complete that degree before you are enrolled in their school.

3. Enroll in a reapplication or specialized post-baccalaureate program.

4. Consider applying to osteopathic medical schools.

5. Apply to one or more foreign medical schools.

6. Seek a career in one of the other allied health professions.

7. You may need to change careers depending on your interests/motivations/or your "application circumstances."

One should consider these options separately, but it is practical to consider a combination of these factors in order to OPTIMIZE one's admission opportunities:

1. REAPPLICATION DURING THE NEXT ACADEMIC YEAR

This may be an appropriate option for those students who received interviews or were "wait-listed." Unfortunately, the majority of re-applicants are still unsuccessful, but if you are attentive to enhancing your resumé/credentials, you have an excellent chance at success. Understanding the reasons why you were unsuccessful the first time around will help you rectify the weaknesses in your application. Make sure you communicate with those schools that interviewed and/or placed you on their waiting list(s). They may provide the necessary information that will be the key to your success.

Depending on the factor(s) that may have affected your first application, you may need to consider the following:

Register at a local college/university/graduate or medical school for science courses that will both enhance your GPA and show that you can succeed at intermediate/ high-level coursework. You should maintain a "B+" to "A" average, an accomplishment that will not be an easy task. (These courses may include physiology, biochemistry, or anatomy and its sub-set of courses such as histology or embryology.)

Work in a clinical/hospital/outpatient setting. This may show that you still have a strong motivation to become a doctor, but it will probably not be the deciding factor in your admission. A part-time or weekend position (paid or volunteer), however, may provide that extra boost for your application.

If your MCATs are a factor, take the time to make the difference. . . . Consider this your mission—TO DO WELL on this exam. . . . Whether you are utilizing commercial prep courses and/or review books, make it your full-time job to do well. If you are reapplying the next academic year, you will have to take the exam that August. That summer you will probably lose most of your free time, but if done properly, you will gain an acceptance letter. If it is necessary that you wait one or more years before applying, use this time to your fullest advantage. . . .   You should be able to master the material without other distractions or time restrictions affecting your performance.

<u>Research level work is another possibility to help build up your credentials</u> .   .   . Remember, however, that coursework and MCAT preparation take precedence if those are the weaker areas.

2.   ENROLL IN A GRADUATE DEGREE PROGRAM

There are a number of graduate school Masters Degree (usually an MS) programs that can be completed in one to two years (usual time is two years) that may give you that "extra boost" for medical school admission. Depending on the academic area, you may even be taking coursework with medical and dental students. Some departmental programs are in or are affiliated with medical schools. Masters Degree programs that are often taught in this manner include biochemistry, physiology, anatomy, microbiology, and pharmacology. Depending on your academic background, masters degrees in other allied health professions (*e.g.* nursing, physical therapy, nutrition) may also be available to you.

If you decide to pursue this pathway, be aware that graduate school is INTENSE. The competition is "stiff" and a "B" average is the minimal expectation. Obtaining a graduate school "B" is much more difficult than that of the undergraduate "B" in the same academic disciplines. If you consider the fact that many other graduate students will be in the medical school applicant pool, graduate students are under intense pressure to do the very best they can. Depending on the graduate school and the program, you may also be expected to finish a masters research project along with a thesis. Most admissions committees require their graduate school applicants to complete their degrees before they enroll in medical school. Leaving graduate school in the middle of your academic program to attend medical school is "not the norm"; if you enroll in a masters degree program, you should expect a one to three year delay before actually enrolling in medical school (with a Ph.D. program it could be five to seven years).

What you will gain if you do enroll in graduate school is personal and intellectual growth, study habits that will help you succeed, and perhaps even a good head start in medical school (e.g. degrees in physiology or biochemistry, etc.). . . . Because graduate school is a big commitment of time, energy, and money, choose a major area that both GENUINELY INTERESTS you and will give you employment opportunities if you are not accepted into medical school. If you do well in graduate school, an admissions committee will have further proof of your motivation, perseverance, and academic abilities.

3.   ENROLL IN A REAPPLICANT OR SPECIALIZED POST-BACCALAUREATE PROGRAM

There are a variety of programs available for applicants who have fulfilled their premedical requirements but who have not applied to medical school or have been previously rejected. By excelling in one of the rigorous programs, the applicant can show that he/she "can do the work" expected in medical school. There is an emphasis on upper division courses which are in the biological sciences and are usually related to medical school studies. Some programs are affiliated with graduate schools/medical schools and award a masters degree after their successful completion. Depending on the school, a research project and thesis may also be required. Other programs do not award a degree but enable the student to schedule those upper division courses which would help the applicant's academic record. Selecting the appropriate coursework (*e.g.* physiology, biochemistry, etc.) would also ease the transition into a medical school curriculum one or two years later.

These programs are rigorous and "B's" and "A's" will be the expectation. Earning a "B" in a graduate school course will obviously be harder than at the college level (Obtaining an "A" will be even more difficult but it can be done!). Medical school admission committees know the hard work and discipline which is necessary to do well in these courses—many of the programs' curricula (except for one or two courses) reflect that of the first year in medical school. Remember that others in your class will also be medical school reapplicants or students who need to strengthen their academic record. You will need to bring your study skills, time-management abilities, and physical, emotional, and mental stamina to a "new higher level." The dividends, however, do eventually pay off; acceptance into medical school and actually knowing the expectations of a first year medical school course level should provide that extra boost for total commitment.

Listed below are descriptions of programs that students may consider before applying/reapplying to medical school:

Master Degree Programs With an Emphasis on Medical School Type Coursework

(Many of the students in these programs are reapplying to medical school. GRE/MCAT scores are submitted as part of the application to the program. Though the programs do not have formal linkages [provisional acceptance into a certain medical school] with medical schools, their acceptance rates can be very impressive.)

DISTRICT OF COLUMBIA

Special Masters Program in Physiology and Biophysics
Department of Physiology and Biophysics
Georgetown University Medical Center
Washington, DC 20007
(202) 687-1179
(202) 687-7407 (FAX)

- One academic year program (Two semesters, thirty-two credit hours).

- Classes taken with medical students.

  1. The grading scale is as follows: letter graded but compared directly with the medical school classes.

  2. MCAT/premedical requirements fulfilled for admission.

  3. Library research project required.

  4. The following courses are taken: microscopic anatomy, embryology, physiology, endocrinology, neuroanatomy, biostatistics/epidemiology.

ILLINOIS

Graduate School Admissions
Applied Physiology Program
Finch University of Health Sciences
The Chicago Medical School
3333 Green Bay Road
North Chicago, IL 60064
(847)578-3209

- Average duration: one year (fall/winter/spring quarters).

- 14-21 credit hours/quarter.

- Programs begin in July.

INDIANA

Preprofessional Non-Thesis M.S. Degree Program
Indiana University—Purdue University at Indianapolis
Department of Biology
723 West Michigan Street
Indianapolis, IN 46202-5132
(317)274-0575
(317)274-2846 (FAX)

- Thirty credit hours, two semester program.

- No thesis.

MASSACHUSETTS

M.A. in Medical Sciences Program
Boston University School of Medicine
Division of Graduate Medical Sciences
715 Albany Street
Boston, MA 02118-2394
(617)638-5120
(617)638-4842 (FAX)

- Program can be completed in twelve months.

- Research/thesis is required.

NEW YORK

Preprofessional M.S. Program
Graduate School of Basic Medical Sciences
New York Medical College
Valhalla, NY 10595
(914)993-4110

- Average duration: two year program.

- Minimum thirty credit hours.

- Evening courses.

- Research (literature review or original project) is required.

- Journal club is offered.

Non-Master Degree Programs

Emphasis is on upper division course work to show both academic excellence and the student's ability to handle a graduate level science curriculum.

CONNECTICUT

Post-Baccalaureate Program
University of Connecticut Health Center School of Medicine
Farmington Avenue
Farmington, CT 06030-1905

- Research opportunity is available.
- Volunteer community service and/or clinical externships are available.

FLORIDA

Premedical Post-Baccalaureate Program
Committee on Premedical Studies
College of Arts and Sciences
University of Miami
PO Box 248004
Coral Gables, FL 33124
(305)284-5176

- Average duration: 1 year.
- Research opportunities and volunteer clinical experiences are available.

PENNSYLVANIA

Post-Baccalaureate Premedical Program
Duquesne University
Suite B-101, Bayer Learning Center
Pittsburgh, PA 15282-1502
(412)396-6335
(412)396-5587 (FAX)

- Volunteer clinical experience is available.

IMS/MSP Programs
Allegheny University of the Health Sciences
Broad and Vine, Room 4122 NCB
Mail Stop 344
Philadelphia, PA 19102-1192

- Allegheny University of the Health Sciences: Medical College of Pennsylvania/ Hahnemann School of Medicine
- Two programs: 1. Interdepartmental Medical Science (IMS)
                2. Medical Science Preparatory (MSP)

1. IMS Program (one year non-degree program)

   • Enrollment in some of the same medical school courses—same exams and grading scales as the first year medical school class.

   • If in good academic standing after the completion of the program, the student has the option to continue studies for one additional year to receive the Master in Medical Science (MMS) degree.

2. MSP Program (one year non-degree program)

   • Designed to help students improve MCAT scores and their academic record.

   • Graduate courses in anatomy, physiology, pharmacology, and biochemistry.

   • Physics and chemistry review courses.

   • MCAT review sessions; mock MCAT exams.

   • Must take the spring MCAT.

   • Participation in community service activity is required.

   • Students have the option of applying to the IMS Program for the following year. The Master in Biological Sciences (MBS) is awarded after successful completion of both programs.

VIRGINIA

Non-Master Degree Program
Premedical Basic Health Services Certificate Program
School of Graduate Studies
Virginia Commonwealth University
Richmond, VA 23284-3051
(804)828-6916

   • Purpose of the program is to enhance one's basic health sciences background.

   • Must have taken the MCAT or GRE.

   • Thirty credit hours of coursework.

   • Two semester program.

   • Must choose one of the following six specialty areas: anatomy, biochemistry, human genetics, microbiology, pharmacology, or physiology.

4.   CONSIDER APPLYING TO OSTEOPATHIC MEDICAL SCHOOLS

Pursuing an osteopathic medical degree (D.O., Doctor of Osteopathy) will give you the same license to practice medicine as your M.D. counterparts. There are 17 D.O. schools nationally where the education requirements are similar to that of allopathic (M.D.) schools. The basic medical sciences occupy the first two years of the curriculum followed by two years of clinical training. Osteopathic medicine's ("osteopathy") philosophy concentrates on the "whole person"/"whole patient"/"whole body" approach—one in which bodily structure and function are interdependently related in the diagnosis and treatment of disease. There is also an emphasis on both the body being good at self-healing and the musculoskeletal system playing a primary role. (Because of the emphasis on the "musculoskeletal system," manipulative medicine is studied and practiced in the osteopathic medical schools).

The majority of osteopathic medical graduates enter primary care residency fields that include family practice, pediatrics, internal medicine, and obstetrics/gynecology. Many osteopaths also do a general internship year before beginning a specialized residency. Osteopathic medicine does have its own structure of residency programs, but there are fewer available positions in many of the specialties (e.g. orthopedics, ophthalmology, dermatology, neurosurgery, cardiovascular surgery, and otolaryngology). If you enter osteopathic medical school and want to eventually enter a non-primary case specialty, be aware that entering those fields will be difficult. Osteopathic medical students are also eligible to take the United States Medical Licensure Examination (USMLE), a series of standardized tests given in the allopathic (M.D.) system. Some osteopathic medical students take these exams (in addition to those given by the National Board of Osteopathic Examiners) to make themselves more competitive if they desire to compete for a M.D. residency position. A number of M.D. residency programs do accept osteopathic graduates—especially if those medical specialties are in primary care. In the most competitive medical (e.g. dermatology) and surgical (e.g. neurosurgery, orthopedics, urology, and otolaryngology) subspecialties, it may be close to impossible for a D.O. to enter an M.D. training program.

Applications to osteopathic medical schools have been steadily rising over the last ten years, making that process also highly competitive. The average admission GPAs and MCAT scores remain lower, however, for osteopathic medical schools when compared to their M.D. counterparts. If you are re-applying to medical school, remember that there are many students who gain admission to an osteopathic medical school after being rejected by M.D. programs.

At the end of this chapter, you will find a list of osteopathic medical school addresses that you can contact for brochures, catalogs, and admissions information. The osteopathic schools use the AACOMAS application service, which is similar to the AMCAS system used by M.D. schools. Additional addresses related to osteopathic medicine are also listed at the end of this chapter.

5. APPLYING TO FOREIGN MEDICAL SCHOOLS (also see Chapter 23, "Foreign Medical Schools")

For some unsuccessful applicants, the desire to be doctors remains so "all encompassing" that they attend foreign medical schools to achieve their dream. There have been many success stories with this option; there have also been many disappointments. The risks involved are quite high. (In some cases, they may even be insurmountable). Some of the schools are run as business enterprises—high tuition and fees paid by hundreds of students with no assurances of a diploma or medical license or opportunity for a U.S. residency; add in a language barrier or limited financial aid opportunities and you could end up stuck in a medical school quagmire!

Although foreign medical schools are discussed in the next chapter, some introductory remarks are in order:

1. United States Governmental Authorities have no accreditation or licensing powers over foreign medical schools. The quality of education can, therefore, rate anywhere from "outright dismal" to "very good."

2. You need to do well on the licensing board exams (USMLE) in order to have a chance at a U.S. residency.

3. Transfers from foreign medical schools into the second or third year of a U.S. medical school occur but are extremely difficult.

4. Some schools advertise that their classes are taught in English. This aspect really applies to the first two years of medical school when the basic sciences are taught. You may still be required to learn (and "not just get by") the native language in order to continue in your clinical years. The hospitals, clinics, and doctors' offices will all use the native language.

5. There may or may not be opportunities for you to do clinical rotations in the U.S. during your third or fourth years.

6. You need to know the financial aid opportunities for each foreign medical school that you are considering in the application process.

7. Be aware of the socioeconomic and political stability of the country you will be living in.

8. An excellent resource for answering your questions about a foreign medical school are U.S. citizen alumni/ae physicians (especially recent graduates from the last few years).

6. ALLIED HEALTH CAREERS/OTHER MEDICALLY RELATED HEALTH CAREERS

This option was introduced in the section on those students considering masters degrees. Many students may not have the academic background to immediately enter such a program (*e.g.* Masters Degree in Physical Therapy; you do not necessarily need a

Bachelors Degree in Physical Therapy (PT) to enter such a program, but you still need appropriate prerequisite coursework). Other unsuccessful medical school applicants may already be nurses, nutritionists, pharmacists, or occupational therapists. Their background gives them a unique opportunity to obtain an advanced degree in their own specialty. There are also other students who seek degrees in accelerated B.S. nursing programs or spend two to three years to receive an additional Bachelors Degree as a Physician's Assistant (P.A.).

Unsuccessful medical school applicants who are allied health professions must still convince a medical school admissions committee why they are changing careers. The initial priorities, as with all unsuccessful applicants, must be to recognize the weaknesses in the prior application, attempt to improve or correct them, and build up one's credentials.

A career change for some unsuccessful applicants may mean seeking a professional degree in another area and becoming a dentist, podiatrist, or chiropractor. If you desire such a degree, you must ask the question: Is this career change or professional degree RIGHT FOR ME?

The amount of time you may need before you reapply to medical school will depend on the weak point(s) of your initial application and your responses for improving or strengthening your credentials. After studying and considering the options, only you can decide which one(s) are appropriate. . . . If you want to become a doctor, then keep the dream alive by persevering and giving "your all" to achieve it! It may take much dedication but the desire to become a physician is a goal directed motivation that for some students CANNOT BE DENIED!

Addresses of Osteopathic Medical Schools

ARIZONA

Office of Admissions
Arizona College of Osteopathic Medicine
Midwestern University
19555 North 59th Avenue
Glendale, AZ 85308
(602) 362-4015

CALIFORNIA

Office of Admissions
Western University of Health Sciences
College of Osteopathic Medicine of the Pacific
College Plaza
Pomona, CA 91766-1889
(909) 623-6116

ILLINOIS

Office of Admissions
Chicago College of Osteopathic Medicine
Midwestern University
555 31st Street
Downers Grove, IL 60515
(800) 458-6253
(630)969-4400

IOWA

Office of Admissions
University of Osteopathic Medicine and
   Health Sciences
College of Osteopathic Medicine and Surgery
3200 Grand Avenue
Des Moines, IA 50312
(515) 271-1450
(515) 271-1578 (FAX)

MISSOURI

Office of Admissions
Kirksville College of Osteopathic Medicine
800 West Jefferson
Kirksville, MO 63501
(800) 626-5266 (ext. 2237)
(816) 626-2237
(816) 626-2969 (FAX)

NEW JERSEY

Admissions Office
University of Medicine and Dentistry
   of New Jersey
School of Osteopathic Medicine Academic
   Center
One Medical Center Drive, Suite 162A
Stratford, NJ 08084
566-7050

(609) 566-6222 (FAX)
NEW YORK
Director of Admissions
New York College of Osteopathic Medicine
of the New York Institute of Technology
Old Westbury, NY 11568
(516) 626-6947
(516) 626-6946 (FAX)

OHIO

Office of Admission
Ohio University
College of Osteopathic Medicine
102 Grosvenor Hall
Athens, OH 45701-2979
(614) 593-4313

OKLAHOMA
Admissions Office
Oklahoma State University
College of Osteopathic Medicine
1111 West 17th Street
Tulsa, OK 74107
(800) 677-1972
(918) 582-1972

PENNSYLVANIA
Office of Admissions
Lake Erie College of Osteopathic Medicine
1858 West Grandview Boulevard
Erie, PA 16509
(814) 866-6641

Assistant Dean for Admissions and
Enrollment Management
Philadelphia College of Osteopathic Medicine
4170 City Avenue
Philadelphia, PA 19131
(800) 999-6998
(215) 871-6719 (FAX)

WEST VIRGINIA
Director of Admissions
West Virginia School of Osteopathic Medicine
400 North Lee Street
Lewisburg, WV 24901
(800) 356-7836 (in WV)
(800) 537-7077 (outside WV)

TEXAS
Office of Medical Student Admissions
University of North Texas Health Science
   Center
Texas College of Osteopathic Medicine
3500 Camp Bowie Boulevard
Fort Worth, TX 76107-2699
(800) 535-TCOM
(817) 735-2204
(817) 735-2225 (FAX)

Additional Information About Osteopathic Medicine

1. The American Osteopathic Association
    142 East Ontario Street
    Chicago, IL 60611
    Telephone: (800) 621-1773, ext. 7401

    Information about: 1. Osteopathic certification and licensing.

                       2. Accredited osteopathic medical schools.

                       3. Accredited osteopathic health care facilities.

                       4. Locating a doctor of osteopathy in your area.

2. The American Academy of Osteopathy
    3500 DePauro Boulevard, Suite 1080
    Indianapolis, IN 46268-1881

    Information about: 1. Osteopathic manipulative treatment (OMT).

                       2. Doctors of Osteopathy who are board certified in OMT.

3. The American Association of Colleges of Osteopathic Medicine (AACOM).
    5550 Friendship Boulevard, Suite 310
    Chevy Chase, MD 20815-4100

    Inquire about the following publications:

    1. *AACOM Organizational Guide.*

    2. *Annual Statistical Report.*

    3. *Application Packet* (no charge).

    4. *College Information Booklet* (brief description of each of the colleges of osteopathic medicine).

    5. *Debts and Career Plans of Osteopathic Medical Students.*

    6. *Osteopathic Medical Evaluation* (single copies of the brochure are free).

23

Foreign Medical Schools

Applying to a foreign medical school(s) should still be considered YOUR LAST OPTION if your career decision is to be a physician. You should "exhaust all other possible options"— even if that means delaying your entry into medical school for one, two, or more years. (For some students going to a foreign medical school is still better than not becoming a doctor at all!) The option of applying to foreign medical schools was first discussed in Chapter 22 ("Knowing the Options If You Are Not Accepted"). That chapter introduced some of the major factors that should concern any applicant seeking a foreign medical degree. Remember that you may spend as much money (or more!) as you would have on a private medical school in the United States and still have no guarantees of even practicing medicine. You should also note that your opportunities regarding the type of residency will also be very limited. Some competitive residency specialties (*e.g.* orthopedics, neurosurgery, ENT, urology, etc.) have United States medical school graduates whom they cannot admit and accommodate!

Major factors (financial aid, language barriers, socioeconomic, and political stability of the country) were first introduced in Chapter 22, but it is important to remind potential applicants that attending a foreign medical school is a very risky endeavor. Language barriers may be insurmountable for some students; though some schools state that their first two years are taught in English, you still need to know the native language for your clinical rotation years. (Another potential problem may be that some basic science faculty members speak English— just not very well!) Some schools offer intensive training in the native language, but learning a new language while you are an adult student in medical school can prove to be extremely difficult. A school's reputation must also be looked at carefully; for example, the granting of fraudulent medical degrees in the Dominican Republic has forced one medical school to close and has hurt the international reputation (especially here in the United States) of the others.

You must also be cautious of agencies that help recruit potential United States applicants for certain foreign medical schools. These organizations usually "market" one or more schools at the same time. There are also foreign medical schools that have "contact" addresses in the United States but that is usually a different situation—these offices are specific for their own school and make it easier for U.S. applicants to find out information and to work through the application bureaucracy.

Remember that the best way to find out information about these schools is through an actual visit: see the facilities, living conditions, meet with U.S. students, and find out information about the faculty, clinical rotations, USMLE passing rates, and the opportunities to return to the United States. Inquiries about these opportunities should include information on the following: 1) The ability to transfer back to a U.S. medical school while still in undergraduate medical training (This is still extremely difficult to do!). 2) Availability of any clinical rotations in the United States during the third or fourth years. 3) Success rates for obtaining an internship/residency in the United States. 4) Requirements for that foreign country's medical degree (*e.g.* Mexico will require a year of internship and then a year of social service [medical] in their country). Some of the United States graduates of Mexican schools are able to obtain a "Fifth Pathway Program"—a year of graduate clinical training at a United States medical school hospital. The Fifth Pathway year substitutes for the internship and social service years that would ordinarily be required. Fifth Pathway Program availability (as to U.S. schools and number of positions) varies on a yearly basis so the United States International Medical Graduate (USIMG) needs to be aware of changes in these programs.

The next section of this chapter summarizes the steps a United States International Medical Graduate must take in order to be eligible for a U.S. medical/surgical residency and the practice of medicine. The last part of this chapter provides a sample list of foreign medical schools where United States applicants have matriculated. Every possible foreign medical school cannot be listed—a separate book could be written about all of the foreign medical schools; the list provides an overview of the opportunities that potentially exist for U.S. applicants. Information on names and addresses of all medical schools in a particular country are usually available from embassy offices. (The embassy addresses are listed for some of the countries.)

Requirements for United States International Medical Graduates to Acquire both a U.S. Residency and the Opportunity to Practice Medicine.

The major step will be to obtain certification by the Educational Commission for Foreign Medical Graduates (ECFMG). Addresses of important offices (including that of the ECFMG) are listed at the end of this section. Certification will include the following steps:

1. The foreign medical school's medical degree will have to be verified directly with the ECFMG; you will also have to prove that you have completed all requirements for that country's M.D. degree. What's more, the medical school must be listed in that year's current edition of the World Directory of Medical Schools (The World Health Organization [WHO] publishes that data).

2. A new requirement will be the passing of an ECFMG Clinical Skills Assessment (CSA) that includes both a test of spoken English (required even if you are a U.S. citizen who speaks fluent English) and a basic medical and clinical science exam. The test taker will need to exhibit mastery of clinical knowledge related to taking a patient's history, physical examination, and the organization and interpretation of clinical data.

3. All parts of the United States Medical Licensing Examination (USMLE) must be passed. Parts I (basic medical sciences) and II (medical school clinical sciences: *e.g.* OB/GYN, Psychiatry, Internal Medicine, Surgery, Pediatrics, Public Health, and Preventive Medicine) are taken during medical school.

4. Part III of the USMLE is taken during your internship/residency training. Part III concerns itself with physician tasks, emergency situations and treatment, initial patient evaluations, and continuing care. There are also a number of questions on outpatient care/ambulatory care treatment.

5. To take Part III of the USMLE, you must have your M.D. degree and have passed Parts I and II. What's more, you must be certified by the ECFMG and have 1-3 years (or more) of a U.S. accredited residency training program.

As you can see, these are the key factors for a United States International Medical Graduate to be able to practice medicine in the U.S. (USIMGs also need to obtain an accredited U.S. residency and fulfill all requirements by the medical licensing board of their particular state.). You can only apply for Part III of the USMLE in the state where you intend to obtain your medical license. Individual states vary in their prerequisite residency training requirements (1-3 years or more) for taking Part III of the USMLE.

The addresses of the individual state boards can be found by contacting the Federation of State Medical Boards (FSMB). The FSMB address is listed in the next section.

List of Important Addresses for U.S. International Medical Graduates

1. United State Medical Licensing Examination
    USMLE
    3750 Market Street
    Philadelphia, PA 19104-3190
    (215) 590-9600

2. Educational Commission for Foreign Medical Graduates
    ECFMG
    3624 Market Street
    Philadelphia, PA 19104-2685
    (215) 386-5900
    (215)386-9196 (FAX)

3. Federation of State Medical Boards
    Federation Place
    400 Fuller Wiser Road, Suite 300
    Euless, Texas 76039-3855
    (817)868-4000

4. National Resident Matching Program (NRMP)
    2501 M Street, NW, Suite 1
    Washington, DC 20037-1307
    (202) 828-0676

Information about the Fifth Pathway Program

    American Medical Association (AMA)
    Licensing and Certification Section
    515 North State Street
    Chicago, IL 60610
    (312) 464-5000

Overview of Foreign Medical Schools

AUSTRALIA

    International Office
    The Flinders University of South Australia
    GPO Box 2100
    Adelaide South Australia 5001
    Toll free from the U.S.: (800) 686-3562
    (up to 25 international students per year)

Queensland and Sydney Universities are also offering spots for international students (including U.S. applicants). These two university medical schools, along with Flinders University, will be sharing a common application form. For more information about these schools, write to the address below (Tell them you are a potential U.S. applicant and would like additional information):

Graduate Medical Admissions
Australian Council for Educational Research (ACER)
Private Bag 55
Camberwell, Victoria, 3124
Australia

CANADA

Of the 16 Canadian medical schools, two have consistently admitted applicants from the United States. The school addresses where you should write for information are listed below:

1. Admissions Office
    Memorial University of Newfoundland
    Faculty of Medicine
    St. John's, Newfoundland
    Canada A1B 3V6
    (709) 737-6615
    (709) 737-5186 (FAX)

2. Admissions Office
    McGill University
    Faculty of Medicine
    3655 Drummond Street
    Montreal, Quebec
    Canada H3G 1Y6
    (514) 398-3517
    (514) 398-4631 (FAX)

    •   The language of instruction is English.

Many Canadian medical schools do not allow foreign applications (including from the U.S.) while others may be considering opening spots in the future for U.S. applicants. All Canadian medical schools are listed and discussed in the annual edition of the AAMC's Medical School Admission Requirements. For more information you should contact the schools directly.

The following addresses are also applicable to Canadian medical schools:

Association of Canadian Medical Colleges
774 Echo Drive
Ottowa, Ontario CANADA K1S 5P2
(613)730-0687
(613)730-1196 (FAX)

Ontario Medical School Application Service (OMSAS)
Ontario Universities' Application Centre
650 Woodlawn Road West
PO Box 1328
Guelph, Ontario CANADA N1H 7P4
(519)823-1940

CARIBBEAN

The Caribbean schools all have English as their official language of instruction. St. George's University School of Medicine in Grenada, West Indies, has had the overall best track record regarding transfers to U.S. schools, clinical rotations in the U.S. and United Kingdom, and also placement in U.S. residencies.

1. St. George's University School of Medicine
    Grenada, West Indies

    United States Contact Office:

    St. George's University School of Medicine
    c/o Medical School Services, Ltd.
    One East Main Street
    Bay Shore, NY 11706-8399
    (800) 899-6337 or
    (516) 665-8500
    (516) 665-5590 (FAX)

2. Ross University
   located in Portsmouth, Dominica

   United States Contact Office:

   > Ross University
   > c/o International Educational Admissions
   > 460 West 34th Street, 12th Floor
   > New York, NY 10001
   > (212) 279-5500
   > (212) 629-3147 (FAX)

3. American University of the Caribbean School of Medicine
   St. Maarten Campus
   174 Defiance Road
   Middle Region
   St. Maarten, Netherlands Antilles

   United States Contact Office:

   > Medical Education Information Office
   > 901 Ponce de Leon Blvd., #201
   > Coral Gables, FL 33134-3036
   > (305) 446-0600

4. SABA University School of Medicine
   PO Box 1000
   Saba, Netherlands Antilles
   011-599-463456
   011-599-463458 (FAX)

   United States Contact Office:
   Education Information Consultants
   PO Box 386
   Gardner, MA 01440
   (508) 630-5122
   (508) 632-2168 (FAX)

IRELAND

The Royal College of Surgeons in Ireland
The Atlantic Bridge Program
10044 Adams Avenue, Suite 302
Huntington Beach, CA 92646
(800) 876-3876 or
(714) 723-6318
(714) 723-4436 (FAX)

- There are twenty-five class positions/year for North American students.

ISRAEL

1. Sackler School of Medicine
   Tel Aviv University
   Ramat Aviv, Israel 69978
   (03) 640-9071

   Contact:

   Sackler School of Medicine
   New York State–American Program
   17 East 62nd Street
   New York, NY 10021
   (212) 688-8811
   (212) 223-0368 (FAX)

   1. Selected candidates are interviewed at the Sackler School of Medicine New York City office (regional interviews can be arranged).
   2. The basic medical sciences are taught in English.
   3. Students can take up to 16 weeks of clinical electives in the United States. Subinternship rotations are also available in the United States.
   4. Knowledge of Hebrew is necessary for the clinical rotations.

2. Faculty of Medicine of the Technion–
   Israel Institute of Technology

   First-year basic medical sciences and training in Hebrew take place in New York (Long Island).

   Contact:

   > The Admissions Office
   > Biomedical Sciences
   > Touro College
   > Building No. 10
   > 135 Carman Road
   > Dix Hills, NY 11746

MEXICO

1. Universidad Autónoma de Guadalajara School of Medicine (UAG)

   United States Office:

   > Universidad Autónoma de Guadalajara
   > Office in the United States
   > 8801 Callaghan Road
   > San Antonio, TX 78230-4414
   > (800) 531-5494 or
   > (210) 366-1611
   > (210) 377-2975 (FAX)

   1. Interviews are only by invitation (either in Guadalajara, Mexico, or San Antonio, Texas).

   2. Two entering classes per year: spring and fall

   3. Intensive Spanish courses are offered.

   4. Fourth year U.S. students can do clinical rotations in UAG's affiliated U.S. hospitals.

   5. The physician's first year after medical school is spent in a rotating internship. This rotating internship is called the "Internado" year (Some Internado spots are available in the United States). The second year after graduation is spent in government-mandated social service (underserved area in medicine).

   6. Six-year program: "Titulo" document is equivalent to the United States M.D. degree (Mexico's Professional Examination must then be passed).

7. Some U.S. graduates of UAG choose to go to the United States through the "Fifth Pathway" program (rotating internship) after finishing the four-year UAG degree. The number of Fifth Pathway spots are limited; after the "Fifth Pathway" year, foreign M.D. graduates enter the National Resident Matching Program (NRMP) for a U.S. residency.

2. Universidad de Monterrey
Coordinadora Curricular de Medicina
Ave. I. Morones Pueto 4500 Pte
C.P. 66238
San Pedro Garza Garcia
Nuevo Leon, Mexico

- Spanish proficiency is required before attending.

PHILIPPINES

Over the years, there have been a number of U.S. citizen alumni from medical schools in the Philippines. A short list of the many schools in the Philippines is listed below:

1. University of the Philippines (Manila)

2. University of the East

3. University of Santo Tomas

4. Manila Central University

5. Far Eastern University

Other Potential Contacts Regarding Foreign Medical Schools

Please note that language barriers may present an insurmountable obstacle to considering attending medical school in Europe. Some medical schools may advertise that they have instruction in English, but the clinical years will require thorough knowledge of the native language (*e.g.* some schools in Hungary [the University Medical School of Pécs] and Poland [1. Karol Marcinkowski University of Medical Sciences in Poznan 2. Jagellonian University School of Medicine in Kraków]). The other European medical schools usually do not offer basic medical sciences taught in English.

If you do seek information from an embassy/consulate, you should state that you are a U.S. citizen who is potentially seeking a position in a medical school of that country.

AUSTRALIA
Embassy of Australia
1601 Massachusetts Avenue, NW
Washington, DC 20036
(800)242-2878 or (202)797-3145
Consulate General
(213)469-4300 (CA) or (415)362-6160
(212)245-4000 (NY)

BELGIUM
Embassy of Belgium
3330 Garfield Street, NW
Washington, DC 20008
(202)333-6900
Consulate General
(213)857-1244 (Los Angeles)
(212)586-5110 (NY)

FRANCE
Embassy of France
4101 Reservoir Road, NW
Washington, DC 20007
(202)944-6200
Consulate General
(310)235-3200 (CA) or (415)397-4330
(212)606-3644 (NY)

GERMANY
Embassy/Federal Republic of Germany
4645 Reservoir Road, NW
Washington, DC 20007
(202)298-4000
Consulate General
(415)775-1061 (CA) or (213)930-2703
(212)308-8700 (NY)

IRELAND
Embassy of Ireland
2234 Massachusetts Avenue, NW
Washington, DC 20008
(202)462-3939
Consulate General
(415)392-4214 (CA)
(212)319-2555 (NY)

ISRAEL
Embassy of Israel
3514 International Drive, NW
Washington, DC 20008
(202)364-5500
Consulate General
(213)852-5500 (CA) or (415)398-8885
(312)565-3300 (IL) or (212)499-5300 (NY)

ITALY
Embassy of Italy
1601 Fuller Street, NW
Washington, DC 20009
(202)328-5500
Consulate General
(310)820-0622 (CA) or
(415)931-4924 (CA)
(212)737-9100 (NY)

MEXICO
Embassy of Mexico
2827 16th Street, NW
Washington, DC 20009-4260
(202)736-1000
Consulate General
(213)351-6800 (CA), (415)392-5554 or
(312)855-1380 (IL)
(212)689-0460 (NY)

PHILIPPINES
Embassy of the Philippines
1600 Massachusetts Avenue, NW
Washington, DC 20036
(202)467-9300
Consulate General
(213)387-5321 (CA) or
(415)433-6666
(212)764-1330 (NY)

POLAND
Embassy of the Republic of Poland
2224 Wyoming Avenue, NW
Washington, DC 20008
(202)232-4517
Consulate General
(310)442-8500 (CA)
(312)337-8166 (IL)
(212)889-8360 (NY)

SPAIN
Embassy of Spain
2375 Pennsylvania Avenue, NW
Washington, DC 20037
(202)42500100

UNITED KINGDOM
British Embassy
19 Observatory Circle, NW
Washington, DC 20008
(202)588-7800
Consulate General
(310)477-3322 (CA)
(312)346-1810 (IL)
(212)745-0200 (NY)

24

Financing Your Medical
School Education

As a successful applicant, you have worked hard to gain admission into medical school. The financial cost of this education, however, will be expensive—you will expend thousands of dollars while also sacrificing several years of income. All of this, however, will be worth it when you reach your professional goal of becoming a doctor. The financing of your medical school education will take careful planning, research, and organization (Yearly tuition can range from less than $5,000 to over $30,000.). This chapter covers a variety of topics related to the financial aid process. As to scholarship, grant, and loan opportunities, it is important to remember that the details (*e.g.* amount loaned or awarded per year, total amount loaned or awarded over four years, interest rate, etc.) of these programs may change during the years you apply and attend medical school. It will be important for you to take the initiative and to stay "up-dated" on this information. (Medical school financial aid offices will be the best sources of information on many of these programs during your educational years.)

Getting Started

If you are requesting financial aid from a federal government-based program, you will need to file the Free Application for Federal Student Aid (FAFSA) form (If you applied for a FAFSA form as an undergraduate, you will now fill out a Renewal form.). Financial aid programs for medical school are designed to help make up the difference between the actual cost of education and the contributions by the individual and his/her family. The contribution by the family is determined using a financial analysis system. (The formula used for calculation is one that is uniform and federally approved. It is periodically reviewed by Congress which then recommends appropriate changes to the financial aid formula.) There are various factors (*e.g.* base-year income, taxes which are paid [federal, state, and local], net value of assets, etc.) and allowances (*e.g.* asset protection, employment allowance, and income protection allowance) that will go into the calculation for evaluating the family contribution. A certain percentage of your assets, for example, will not go into the calculation because they are considered "protected" for your future retirement.

It is not a requirement to supply information about parental income when you are filing the FAFSA form for loan programs funded through the Department of Education. This option regarding parental income applies to such programs as Federal Stafford Loans and Federal Perkins Loans. For those programs, the medical student is considered "independent" and parental income is not used in the calculations to determine "monetary need."

You should know, however, that medical schools will still consider their students to be "dependent" and will ask that the parents' financial information be disclosed. You may be given the option not to provide this information to the individual medical school; you should be aware, however, that most schools will make their need-based financial aid awards according to the financial information of the student (and spouse) and his/her parents. Medical schools also administer their own scholarship, grant, and loan programs and want to make sure that the funds are properly distributed (There is an expectation that families should contribute to the financing of the student's medical education.).

If a student wants to be considered for a medical school's financial aid program, he/she should follow the guidelines/suggestions of that institution. Medical schools will, of course, take into account various circumstances that may affect your financial aid award. You may, for example, have one or more siblings attending college and that circumstance would directly affect your parents' contribution to your medical education. (It will then be necessary to "verify" that information; the medical school financial aid office will provide enrollment verification forms that need to be signed by the college(s) attended by your sibling(s).) If a student's parents are divorced, financial aid offices will still expect to have documentation regarding their individual incomes so that a contribution assessment can be made.

The financial office at your medical school will also want you to inform them of any change in financial circumstances. Whether you are entering medical school as a first- year student or are already enrolled, it will be very important to formally report any changes. Examples may include a change in marital status, parental income, or additional scholarship aid (from another source). A medical school's guidelines regarding a change in financial status are extremely important to follow—if a student does not report these changes, he/she could lose the scholarship grant, or loan, or could have an award reversed—one which was given in a previous semester.

Budgets

As an aspiring medical student, you should be aware that your proposed "personal budget" for the school year will vary with that of the budget used for purposes of applying for financial aid. Your financial aid award will usually be based on a number of basic parameters which include the following: (NOTE: There are a number of factors which are excluded in financial aid evaluation which you nonetheless will have to consider. . . . They are discussed in the next section.).

Basic Medical School Educational Expense Budget

1. TUITION

2. STUDENT FEES

3. LIVING EXPENSES (ROOM AND BOARD)

4. BOOKS

5. EQUIPMENT/SUPPLIES

6. TRANSPORTATION

7. PERSONAL EXPENSES (*e.g.* CLOTHING, LAUNDRY, RECREATION, EXPENSES FOR BASIC DENTAL CARE, ETC.)

The medical school's financial aid office will provide you with an estimated educational expense budget for a first-year entering student. As you progress in your medical school career, there will be additional expenses that will have to be considered—your transportation costs will increase as you travel to various hospitals for your clinical rotations. Your living and personal expenses will also increase because your schedule will be longer than the regular pre-clinical academic years.

As a student, you really should consider each of these factors which will account for a medical school's estimated educational cost. Tuition will obviously vary according to whether the school is a private or public institution (depending on the state, there are some "tuition bargains" if you happen to be a resident attending a public institution). If you are an out-of-state resident attending a public medical school, your tuition costs will be higher. If you fit into this category, you should plan on paying this tuition rate for a minimum of one year. It will be your decision and responsibility to fulfill the necessary requirements to establish residency in a new state. As for tuition, every applicant should inquire about any estimated tuition hikes over the next one to two years.

School fees will also be a fixed cost for that academic year. You should know exactly what you are paying for and the medical school will provide you with a list of these costs. These fees vary at each school and may include some of the following: student government/associations/organizations, athletic/recreational, health insurance premium (If you are not covered by a parent's/spouse's health plan, you can enroll in a university plan and pay the appropriate premium.), library and/or publication fees, etc. Some schools may also include examination fees (USMLE). The passing of various parts of this test is required by many schools before students can continue their medical school studies.

During your first two years of medical school, you will be required to purchase or rent different types of medical instruments (*e.g.* stethoscope) or equipment (*e.g.* microscope). This factor will also be listed separately as an educational cost and an estimate will be provided by the medical school.

Books and supplies will also be factored into the budget. This factor is usually based on a "reasonable cost"—a medical student simply cannot purchase every book on a course list. There are, however, those books that will be required for the course. "Personal allowance" costs will also be provided and will vary with the particular medical school. Personal expenses may include, for example, a reasonable allowance for clothing, recreation, laundry, etc. (It will not include that warm-weather spring break vacation you may want to take!). When comparing medical school costs (tuition, fees, etc.), you should also look closely at this category to see what areas are covered and the monetary allowance that is provided.

If you have an automobile, your car insurance payments should be secured under the transportation allowance. (Purchasing an automobile and then making monthly payments would not be covered by the cost allowance.) Depending on the school, expenses for fuel, parking, tolls, bus fares, and automobile repairs may be budgeted under transportation or personal expenses or may have their own category.

Room and board expenses will vary according to the location of the school (large city, medium-size or small city/town). Many medical students live off-campus while some utilize university housing (if available). Some schools encourage their students to live on-campus (especially if there are an adequate number of dorms or apartments allotted for medical students) and base the living expense allowance according to on-campus costs. If you attend a school of this type and live off-campus, the financial aid office may require you to document that you could not obtain on-campus housing. This will be necessary so that any loan allowance can cover living off-campus.

There may also be other items that you may need to consider in your budget (An allowance for them will depend on the individual medical school.). A few examples would include child care expenses/dependent care allowance, uninsured medical and dental expenses (health care costs which are not covered by your insurance plan(s)) and life insurance. If you are a married student or single parent, the cost of life insurance may be approved when considering your final budget.

As you further plan your educational budget, you should be aware of some of the expenses that a medical school cannot include in determining your financial aid package (There are federal government rules and guidelines which schools must follow.). Some examples of expenses that are not permitted in a cost budget allowance are listed on the following page.

Examples of Items That Are Not Included in a School's Estimated Cost Budget Allowance

1. CONSUMER DEBTS

   (*e.g.* commercial credit cards, department store credit cards, etc.)

2. THE PURCHASE OF AN AUTOMOBILE

3. RELOCATION EXPENSES

   (NOTE: Moving to your new medical school will undoubtedly add an expense to your first budget that will not be covered by a financial aid loan or grant program.)

4. EQUIPMENT THAT IS "OPTIONAL"

   The most common example is a personal computer. Though the use of a computer is very common these days, the cost of such equipment will not be considered for "budgeting purposes" unless it is a requirement that all students have this piece of equipment. (NOTE: A "requirement" of this type would be highly "unlikely." Most medical schools, for example, have computer labs which are accessible to the student body for personal use.)

5. INTERNSHIP/RESIDENCY INTERVIEW EXPENSES

   You will incur these additional expenses as a fourth year medical student. Depending on the number of applications and the location of your prospective hospitals, you may incur a considerable expense for application and traveling/interview expenses.

6. CLINICAL ROTATIONS AWAY FROM YOUR MEDICAL SCHOOL

   Some students choose to do out-of-town electives in their fourth year. Many choose rotations at hospitals where they are considering a potential residency application (and hopefully an interview). This is a sound investment for one's professional future but the medical student will be expected to pay for the costs (travel/living expenses) of those rotations.

   Remember to read over all financial aid application forms (FAFSA and the individual medical schools) so that all information will be entered correctly; pay close attention to those items that are excluded from the budget analysis—they may be excluded for financial aid purposes but you must still take them into account for your "personal budget." In trying to set up your budget, it is important to keep in mind many of the individual factors that will be part of it. The following detailed list should help get you started for both the first year of medical school and "beyond" (including the "clinical years").

Sample Items for a Medical Student Budget

INCOME/ASSETS/LOANS

1. Personal Contribution

    - Savings
    - Summer income
    - Other potential assets (stocks, bonds, etc.)

2. Parental/Spousal Contribution

3. Scholarships/Grants

    - Medical school-based aid
    - Outside resources (*e.g.* organizations, associations, and private foundations)
    - Government programs

4. Loans

    - Federal government-based aid
    - Medical school-based aid
    - Banks
    - Other loan programs
    - Personal loans

5. Other (*e.g.* Military)

EXPENSES

1. Tuition

2. Additional Medical Student Fees

3. Books and Supplies

4. Medical Instruments/Equipment/Lab Coats

5. Transportation
    1. Automobile
        - insurance
        - car payments
        - fuel

- repairs/maintenance
- parking
- tolls

2. Public Transportation
   - fares

3. Other Travel Expenses
   - vacations
   - residency interviews

6. Food
   - groceries
   - school cafeteria menu plans
   - hospital cafeteria costs

7. Rent/Mortgage Payments

8. Utilities

9. Household Furniture/Furnishings/Repairs

10. Child Care Expenses

11. Clothing Purchases/Laundry

12. Other Personal Items

13. Credit Card Payments

14. Examination Fees (USMLE Parts I and II)

15. Relocation Expenses

16. Internship/Residency Application and Interviewing Expenses

17. Clinical Rotations Away From Your Medical School

18. Insurance
    - health
    - life
    - automobile
    - renters/homeowners
    - disability
    - fire

20. Medical/Dental/Optical
    - expenses not covered by insurance

Helpful Hints When Applying for Financial Aid

1. You should maintain a good credit rating. Obtaining your initial loans and then applying for additional ones over the next few years will require you to maintain an acceptable credit rating.

2. Read and understand the details of all financial aid information pamphlets and applications. Remember that loan programs may change and it will be important to keep updated on this information. Making sure you understand the details of the loan agreement(s) will also help you to plan your financial future—information on such factors as deferments, grace periods, and repayment schedules are all very important. You should also know the meaning of the various financial terms used in loan agreements (*e.g.* amortization, deferred interest, graduated repayment, loan consolidation, etc.). Many lenders provide direct information (*e.g.* booklets, pamphlets, etc.) to their borrowers to help them understand this terminology.

3. Remember to start the financial aid application process (*e.g.* FAFSA form) before you are accepted into medical school. You should also begin to research outside (*e.g.* non-government or non-school based aid) scholarship and grant opportunities. It will also be necessary for you to find out appropriate information about financial aid programs (*e.g.* government and school-based aid) at particular medical schools.

4. Meet all deadlines for sending in financial aid applications and other supporting documents.

5. Your financial information must be accurate and correct. You should be able to document or verify any financial information/data you put into an application.

6. If there are any corrections, changes, or updates with your financial status, you should inform all of the appropriate offices (*e.g.* financial aid office, banks, government agencies, etc.).

7. Keep copies of all of your important documents, agreements, letters, etc. in a separate financial aid file. You need to keep all of this information well-organized so that you can refer to it as needed during the school year or in the future.

8. It will be very important to formulate a budget for your medical school years. As seen in the first part of this chapter, the cost of medical school is more than "tuition, room and board;" keep all of these extra cost factors in mind—they can add up quickly and you need to be aware of them so that you can accurately determine your personal budget.

9. Your parents and/or spouse will also have to be directly involved in the financial aid process. If you are seeking a financial need-based scholarship/loan, it will be necessary for such family members to submit financial information.

10. Make sure that you inquire about any expected tuition rate hikes over the next one to two years. The " cost of living" factor will also be a key issue in your budgeting process—your medical school, along with students, can be good resources for information regarding this aspect of your personal budget.

11. You need to have excellent skills at "debt management." Medical school is an expensive but very worthwhile and rewarding investment—taking that first loan out will be the beginning of a time frame when you will "run a personal monetary deficit;" you need, however, to take control of your debt—"runaway spending" must be avoided at all costs! You will soon be an intern/resident—repayment periods come sooner than you think!

12. "Debt management" involves many factors, but you must learn to live within a budget. . . Delayed gratification again becomes a major theme but you must remember that you are making a large personal investment in your professional future. Over the years, medical students have practiced a "myriad of common-sense methods" to cut back on personal costs If you do the simple things—car-pooling, sharing rent, packing a lunch, eating dinner at home (or signing on to a university cafeteria food plan)—the end result will be a savings of hundreds or even thousands of dollars. What will you do with that money? . . . Your debt management skills should guide you to the right decision!

Student Rights and Responsibilities

As a consumer/student borrower, you must know your rights and responsibilities. There are numerous federal guidelines and regulations that are followed by financial aid offices and lenders which provide a "framework of protection" for the consumer; at the same time, however, there are the responsibilities of the borrower which must be taken very seriously.

A summary of some of these rights and responsibilities are listed below:

STUDENT RIGHTS

As a student, you have the right to know:

• What financial aid programs are available.

- The application deadlines for each of these available programs.

- How financial need is determined (*e.g.* costs for tuition, fees, room and board, books/supplies, personal expenses, etc.) and how these factors relate to an educational budget.

- How much of this financial need will be covered by loan and by grants/scholarship funding.

- What sources (*e.g.* your assets, parents' contribution, etc.) are utilized in determining your financial need.

- How the financial aid will be distributed.

- You can request an explanation of the various programs in your financial aid package.

- The financial details of the loan agreement. Some of these factors may include:

    1. The total amount that must by repaid.

    2. Interest rate.

    3. The length of time to repay the loan.

    4. When you must start repaying the loan.

    5. Minimum repayment amounts.

    6. List of any charges/fees (*e.g.* loan origination fee) and how they are collected.

    7. Available options for refinancing or consolidating the loan(s).

    8. The ability to prepay the loan without any "prepayment penalties."

    9. An explanation of "defaulting on a loan" and its consequences to you as a consumer.

    10. Grace and deferment periods; loan forbearance.

- The yearly amounts that you can receive from the various programs.

- The total amounts that can be loaned during your medical school years.

- You will have an "entrance counseling session" before you receive your first loan disbursement. Before you leave medical school, you will receive "exit counseling." These sessions will provide very important information about your loan.

- How your medical school determines "satisfactory" academic progress and what happens if you are not achieving this standard.

EXAMPLES OF STUDENT RESPONSIBILITIES

- You must read all information provided by the financial aid office and the lending institutions. (If there are details that you do not understand—ask the appropriate questions!)

- You need to carefully read and understand all financial agreements/contracts that you are asked to sign. (Again, you should ask questions about information that is ambiguous or that you do not understand.) You should also keep copies of these documents.

- Complete all application forms as indicated. If there are requests for the additional documents, you should respond promptly.

- If there are any corrections (or new information/additions), make them in a timely manner.

- Complete all documents on time—you need to meet all application and loan agreement deadlines.

- Correct information is essential. Misreporting information could subject you to penalties under federal law.

- Understand the school's refund policy regarding such student status changes as withdrawal, leaves of absence, or dismissal.

- Notify all appropriate parties (*e.g.* school, lender agency, etc.) if there is any type of change in your school attendance status.

- Know the medical school's standards for satisfactory academic progress.

- You must attend an entrance counseling session before you receive your first money disbursement. When you leave medical school, you must attend an exit counseling session.

- Be aware of the requirements/financial terms of the agreement—you have signed a legal document and are responsible for repayment.

- Be aware of all time periods (*e.g.* grace and deferment periods) that may affect your repayment schedule.

Loan, Grant, and Scholarship Programs

The remaining parts of this chapter provide information on a variety of financial aid programs. These sections are divided in the following manner:

- Federal Loan Programs
- Other Loan Programs
- Special Federal Grant Programs
- Armed Services Scholarship Programs
- National Health Service Corps Scholarship Program/Qualified Loan Repayment Program
- Special Scholarship, Grant, and Loan Programs (Contact Addresses)
- Other Financial Aid Possibilities
- Research Fellowships and Other Awards for Medical Students

Federal Loan Programs

1. FEDERAL STAFFORD LOAN (SUBSIDIZED)

   - The student must show financial need to qualify for the loan.

   - Must be a United States citizen, a U.S. National, or a permanent resident of the U.S.

   - The annual maximum loan limit is $8,500. The cumulative total for undergraduate studies and medical school is $65,500.

   - A variable interest rate is applied which is not to exceed 8.25 percent. This rate is based on a 91-day Treasury Bill (T-Bill) plus 2.5 percent (while in school, grace and deferment periods). During the repayment period, the interest rate is based on a 91-day T-Bill plus 3.1 percent.

   - The federal government pays the loan interest while the student is in medical school (and during grace/deferment periods).

   - Banks, credit unions, eligible schools, and the federal government are the lending institutions for this loan.

   - Disbursement of funds can be through the medical school. The university receives the funds from the Department of Education.

   - Grace period for loan repayment lasts for 6 months after graduation. Interest is then charged directly to the borrower after the grace period ends.

   - No deferment is allowed during residency for new borrowers of these funds (after 7/1/93). Loan repayment forbearance is available (*e.g.* economic hardship).

   - Repayment period: usually up to 10 years.

   - There are no prepayment penalties.

   - The student is permitted to consolidate this loan.

2. FEDERAL STAFFORD LOAN (UNSUBSIDIZED)

   - The student does not have to demonstrate financial need. Cost of medical school attendance, however, is an important factor for loan eligibility.

   - The student must be a United States citizen, a U.S. National, or a U.S. permanent resident.

   - Banks, credit unions, eligible schools, and the federal government are the lending institutions for this loan.

   - Annual maximum unsubsidized loan limit is $10,000. (The total Stafford Loan limit is $18,500—of this amount, $8,500 would be allowed as the "subsidized" amount.)

   - The cumulative loan total for undergraduate and medical school studies is $138,500 (total amount for both subsidized and unsubsidized Stafford loans).

- A variable interest rate is applied and is based on a 91-day T-Bill plus 2.5 percent (while in school and during grace and deferment periods). During the repayment period, the interest rate is based on a 91-day T-Bill plus 3.1 percent.

- The total interest rate is not to exceed 8.25 percent.

- Interest on the loan does accumulate while in school and during grace and deferment periods. The student is later responsible for paying the interest amount which accumulates.

- A grace period for loan repayments lasts for 6 months after graduation.

- No deferment is allowed during residency (Loan forbearance is available [*e.g.* economic hardship]).

- Repayment period: normally up to 10 years.

- There are no penalties for prepayment of the loan.

- The student is permitted to consolidate this loan.

3. FEDERAL PERKINS LOAN

- The student must demonstrate financial need.

- The loan program is sponsored by the federal government but the medical ochool administers the funds

- The student must be a United States citizen, U.S. National, or a U.S. permanent resident.

- Annual maximum loan limit is $5,000. The aggregate loan total for both undergraduate and medical school studies is $30,000.

- A 5 percent interest rate is applied to the loan.

- No interest is charged directly to the borrower while in medical school or during deferment or grace periods. Interest is charged to the borrower after the grace period has expired.

- Grace period is for 9 months after graduation.

- No deferment is allowed during residency. Forbearance may be available for appropriate circumstances (*e.g.* economic hardship).

- Repayment period is up to 10 years.

- There are no penalties for prepayment of the loan.

- The student is permitted to consolidate this loan.

4. PRIMARY CARE LOAN

- The loan is considered a medical school campus-based loan but the sponsor is the Department of Health and Human Services.

- Must be a U.S. citizen, U.S. National, or a U.S. permanent resident.

- The student must show financial need, and parental income/asset information must be provided on the FAFSA form.

- As part of the loan contract, the student must agree to enter and finish a complete residency in primary care and practice in that primary care specialty (until he/she repays the loan in full).

- Students may borrow funds which cover tuition plus an additional $2,500. There is no limit on the total cumulative amount (This, of course, relates to the student's tuition cost).

- The interest rate is 5 percent. If the student /physician does not meet the primary care agreement (during the time period before the loan is completely repaid), the interest rate will increase to 12 percent/year (It will be compounded annually from the date of the loan issuance.). The borrower will also be required to repay the loan in full no longer than three years from the day on which he/she failed to comply with the primary care agreement.

- No interest accumulates for the borrower while in medical school or during grace or deferment periods. Interest is charged to the borrower only after grace/deferment periods are completed.

- Grace period is for 12 months after graduation from medical school.

- A deferment is allowed during the primary care residency.

- The repayment period is up to 10 years.

Other Loan Programs

The Association of American Medical Colleges sponsors the MEDLOANS℠ Program which is designed for students attending allopathic medical schools. Student access to the Federal Stafford Loan Programs (subsidized and unsubsidized) can also be obtained through this AAMC program. MEDLOANS also offers the Alternative Loan Program (ALP) and the MEDEX Loan Program. The MEDEX program provides loans for fourth year medical students to help cover residency interview and relocation costs (Medical school and other financial aid programs do not allow for these expenses.). A brief summary of the Alternative Loan Program (ALP) is provided on the next page:

ALTERNATIVE LOAN PROGRAM (ALP)

- Sponsored by the AAMC MEDLOANS℠ Program. The lender is the Household Bank (Indianapolis, IN).

- Helps supplement other loan programs utilized by the student.

- The student must be a U.S. citizen and be a full-time student at an accredited allopathic U.S. medical school.

- The student must be in satisfactory academic standing, have an adequate credit rating, and cannot be in default on any other loans.

- Minimum annual amount is $500. Cumulative/aggregate amount is $175,000.

- Variable interest rate is applied; during medical school, the rate of the 91-day T-Bill plus 2.5 percent is applied. After graduation, the rate of the 91-day T-Bill plus 2.85 percent is applied.

- No prepayment penalties.

- Deferment is up to 3 years after graduation.

- Loan repayment: up to 20 years.

- More information on this program can be obtained by calling (800) 858-5050 or writing the Association of American Medical Colleges, MEDLOANS Program, 2450 N Street, NW, Washington, DC 20078-6732.

Special Federal Grant Programs

1. FADHPS PROGRAM: FINANCIAL ASSISTANCE FOR DISADVANTAGED HEALTH PROFESSIONS STUDENTS

   - Sponsored by the U.S. Department of Health and Human Services.

   - Students must be from a disadvantaged background and be of exceptional financial need. They must also be a U.S. citizen, a U.S. National, or a U.S. permanent resident.

   - Parental income/asset information is required on the FAFSA form.

   - The award is based upon need. The yearly contribution by the family cannot exceed the lesser of $5,000 or one-half the cost of one's medical school education.

   - Students should obtain information directly from the financial aid office at the medical schools (allopathic and osteopathic) that participate in this program.

   - Scholarships are dependent upon annual funding. Grants are awarded to cover tuition and other reasonable educational costs (up to $10,000).

- In exchange for financial support, students must agree to enter and complete training in a primary care specialty (*e.g.* general internal medicine, family practice, general pediatrics, and public health/preventative medicine) and practice in that specialty for five years after completing the residency training program. The student/physician must enter this residency program no longer than four years after medical school graduation.

- If the physician fails to enter and practice primary health care medicine for the specific time period, a penalty will be assessed. This includes repayment of all scholarship funds received under the agreement that was previously entered (at the maximum prevailing interest rate which is determined by the Treasury Department).

2. EXCEPTIONAL FINANCIAL NEED (EFN) PROGRAM

- Sponsored by the U.S. Department of Health and Human Services.

- The award is based upon need. The yearly contribution by the family cannot exceed the lesser of $5,000 or one-half the cost of one's medical school education.

- Scholarships are dependent upon annual funding. Maximum award: tuition/fees/appropriate educational expenses.

- Parental income/asset information is required on the FAFSA form.

- Eligibility (primary care training and practice) and penalty terms are applicable—see previous descriptions of these same areas under the FADHPS Program.

Armed Services Scholarship Programs

These scholarship programs are highly competitive and are awarded by the Army, Air Force, and Navy. Students receive funding (*e.g.* tuition, books/supplies, monthly stipend, authorized fees) for their medical education but must serve one year of active duty for each year of support that is provided. Some physicians will be able to serve their residency training programs at a military hospital/facility. It should be noted, however, that this time will not substitute for the service obligation owed to the military. A brief overview of these programs is provided below:

1. ARMED FORCES HEALTH PROFESSIONS SCHOLARSHIP: UNITED STATES ARMY

- Must be a U.S. citizen.

- Student must be enrolled or have an acceptance letter from an accredited medical school (allopathic or osteopathic) in the United States or Puerto Rico.

- Meet all other prescribed eligibility criteria for an appointment as a commissioned officer.

- Covers tuition and other certain required expenses.

- The student enters the program as a commissioned officer in the United States Army Reserve and during school receives a stipend for ten and one-half months each year. For the remaining time (active duty training), the student receives pay and allowances as a Second Lieutenant.

- As a scholarship participant, the student will be required to apply for the Army's first year graduate medical education program. If the student is not selected, he/she can complete that part of the training (internship and/or residency) in a civilian hospital (active duty will be delayed during the time that is spent training in a civilian hospital).

- Further information can be obtained by contacting your local/regional Army recruiter or by contacting the following address: U.S. Army Health Professions Support Agency SGPS-PD, 5109 Leesburg Pike, Falls Church, VA 22041-3258.

2. ARMED FORCES HEALTH PROFESSIONS SCHOLARSHIP: U.S. NAVY

- Must be a U.S. citizen.

- Student must be enrolled or have an acceptance letter from an accredited medical school (allopathic or osteopathic) in the United States or Puerto Rico.

- Must meet all other prescribed eligibility criteria for an appointment as a commissioned officer.

- Commission as an ensign in the United States Naval Reserve.

- Tuition, authorized fees, reimbursement for approved books and supplies that are required purchases.

- Receive a stipend for ten and one-half months each year and their full-duty pay for 45 days (active duty training) each year.

- Students will be required to apply for an internship in a naval hospital. If the student is not selected, he/she can complete that part of the training (internship and/or residency) in a civilian hospital (Active duty will be delayed during the time that is spent training in a civilian facility.).

- Further information can be obtained by contacting your local/regional Navy recruiter or by contacting the following address: Navy Recruiting Command (Code 32), 801 North Randolph Street, Arlington, VA 22203-1991.

3. AIR FORCE HEALTH PROFESSIONS SCHOLARSHIP PROGRAM

    *   Must be a U.S. citizen.

    *   The applicant must be accepted to an accredited U.S. medical school with a minimum MCAT score of 24.

    *   Must meet all other prescribed eligibility criteria for an appointment as a commissioned officer (Second Lieutenant in the Air Force Reserve.).

    *   The student must be commissioned prior to his/her 35th birthday.

    *   Tuition, fees, and books.

    *   Monthly stipend.

    *   45 days of active duty each summer. During active duty, the student gets full pay as a Second Lieutenant.

    *   Opportunity for postgraduate education.

    *   Further information may be obtained by contacting your local/regional Air Force recruiter or by contacting the following address: Medical Recruiting Division HQ, USAFRS/RSOHM, 550 D Street West, Suite 1, Randolph AFB, TX 78150-4527.

National Health Service Corps Scholarship Program/ Loan Repayment Program

The National Health Service Corps is a component of the Health Resources and Services Administration, an agency of the U.S. Public Health Service. Under this program, the Bureau of Primary Health Care provides scholarships to medical students who agree to serve in a federally designated health professional shortage area. A brief summary of this program is as follows:

1. NATIONAL HEALTH SERVICE CORPS SCHOLARSHIP PROGRAM

    *   Bureau of Primary Health Care.

    *   U.S. citizens or Nationals who are accepted or enrolled in an accredited (allopathic or osteopathic) U.S. medical school.

    *   Scholarship benefits include: tuition and fees, other reasonable educational expenses (*e.g.* payment towards supplies and books), and a monthly stipend.

    *   Approved primary care specialties include: general internal medicine, general pediatrics, family practice, and obstetrics and gynecology.

    *   One year of service is required for each year of scholarship support.

- There is a minimum two-year obligation.

- Physicians are required to practice medicine in federally designated high-priority health professional shortage areas (HPSA). These sites are approved by the Public Health Service.

- More information can be obtained by contacting:

Bureau of Primary Health Care
National Health Service Corps
Scholarship Program
4350 East West Highway
10th Floor
Bethesda, MD 20814
(800)638-0824

2. QUALIFIED LOAN REPAYMENT PROGRAM

- National Health Service Corps/U.S. Public Health Service.

- Funds provided for loan repayment.

- Payment of up to $25,000 per year for two years of service commitment; up to $35,000 per year (at qualifying sites) beyond a two-year period.

- Additional payments to help with tax liabilities incurred from having your loan repaid.

- Minimum service commitment: two years.

- Eligible specialties include family medicine, general pediatrics, general internal medicine, obstetrics/gynecology, or general psychiatry.

- Physicians must practice in a facility/geographic area designated by the National Health Services Corps/U.S. Public Health Service.

- The Physician also receives a salary and other basic benefits.

- More information can be obtained by contacting:

National Health Service Corps
ATTN: Loan Repayment Programs
2070 Chain Bridge Road
Suite 450
Vienna, VA 22182
(800)221-9393

Special Scholarship, Grant, and Loan Programs
(Contact Addresses)

Financial Resources For Women:

American Association of University Women (AAUW)
Educational Foundation
2201 North Dodge Street
PO Box 4030
Iowa City, IA 52243-4030
(319)337-1716
(319)337-1204 (FAX)

Business and Professional Women's Foundation Scholarship Program
2012 Massachusetts Avenue, NW
Washington, DC 20036

American Medical Women's Association (AMWA)
Medical Education Loan Program
800 North Fairfax Street
Suite 400
Alexandria, VA 22314
(703)838-0500
(703)549-3864

Financial Resources For Minority Group Members:

National Medical Fellowships, Inc.
ATTN: Executive Secretary
254 West 31st Street, 7th Floor
New York, NY 10001
(212)714-0933

- American Indian, African-American, Mexican American and Mainland Puerto Rican students.

Emergency Scholarships for American Indian Students
Association on American Indian Affairs
245 5th Avenue, Suite 1801
New York, NY 10016
(212)689-8720

Bureau of Indian Affairs for American Indians and Eskimos
ATTN: Director of Higher
Education Programs
PO Box 26567
615 First Street, NW
Albuquerque, NM 87125

Other Financial Aid Possibilities

1. Medical School Based Aid (*e.g.* scholarships, grants, loans)

    *   Make inquiries at your medical school about these possibilities.

2. Loan Forgiveness and Repayment Programs (*e.g.* state-based aid; inquire at your medical school). This usually involves a service obligation—many times in one of the primary care specialties. Your medical school should have information about these programs.

3. Programs sponsored by various groups and organizations:
    *   Women's organizations
    *   Fraternal organizations
    *   Employers (applicant's or parent's)
    *   Ethnic groups
    *   Veterans associated organizations
    *   County/state medical societies
    *   Church groups/religious organizations

Research Fellowships/Awards for Medical Students

Listed below are a variety of opportunities for medical students to do both original research and to receive stipends for their work. Depending on the fellowship, these programs may be as short as two or three months (There are a variety of summer programs.) or may extend to one year. These awards are usually based on the specific basic medical science/clinical discipline that is being researched. (Because the details [*e.g.* eligibility requirements, stipends, travel allowances, application deadlines, etc.] of these programs may change from year to year, only the contact addresses and telephone numbers are listed.) It is important to make inquiries in the early part of the academic year—information and applications will then be sent directly to you, providing you with sufficient time to prepare a research proposal (if applicable). Many of these programs require you to have a faculty sponsor/mentor in order to be eligible for the fellowship. A few programs allow the student to do research at an assigned laboratory (usually at the research facility where the fellowship is sponsored).

Those programs marked with an asterisk (*) are the ones which have the student travel to their clinical/research site for the duration of the fellowship.

ALLERGY, ASTHMA, IMMUNOLOGY

American Academy of Allergy, Asthma,
  and Immunology
ATTN: Summer Fellowships
611 East Wells Street
Milwaukee, WI 53202
(414)272-6071
(414)272-6070 (FAX)

DIABETES

Vanderbilt Diabetes Research and Training
  Center
ATTN: Summer Student Research Program
Vanderbilt University School of Medicine
Nashville, TN 37232-0615
(615)322-7001
(615)343-0490 (FAX)

GASTROENTEROLOGY

Research and Education Department
Crohn's and Colitis Foundation
  of America
Student Research Fellowship Awards
386 Park Avenue South
New York, NY 10016
(800)932-2423 or
(212)685-3440
(212)779-4098 (FAX)

MEDICAL HISTORY/MEDICAL HUMANISM

Osler Society
Student Research Award
c/o Center for Perinatal Biology
Loma Linda University School of Medicine
Loma Linda, CA 92350
(909)824-4325

MEDICAL RESEARCH (various specialties)

National Student Research Forum
University of Texas Medical Branch
301 University Boulevard
Galveston, TX 77555-1317
(409)772-3763

NEUROLOGY

American Academy of Neurology
ATTN: Essay Award Contest
1080 Montreal Avenue
ST. Paul, MN 55116
(612)695-1940

Epilepsy Foundation of America National
  Office
ATTN: Health Sciences Student Fellowship
4351 Garden City Drive
Landover, MD 20785-2267

Parkinson's Disease Foundation
ATTN: Medical Student Fellowships
William Black Medical Research Building
Columbia—Presbyterian Medical Center
710 West 168th Street
New York, NY 10032
(800)457-6676 or
(212)923-4700

NEUROSURGERY

Barrow Neurological Institute
ATTN: Medical Student Clerkships
350 West Thomas Road
Phoenix, AZ 85013-4496
(602)285-3000

NUCLEAR MEDICINE

Society of Nuclear Medicine
Education and Research Foundation
ATTN: Student Fellowship Award
1850 Samuel Morse Drive
Reston, VA 20190-5316
(703)708-9000
(703)708-9015 (FAX)

NUTRITION

American Society of Clinical Nutrition
National Clinical Nutrition Internship
9650 Rockville Pike
Bethesda, MD 20814-3998
(301)530-7110
(301)571-1863 (FAX)

ONCOLOGY

Summer Oncology Research Program
Roswell Park Cancer Institute
Elm and Carlton Streets
Buffalo, NY 14263
(716)845-2339

OPHTHALMOLOGY

Prevent Blindness America
Fight for Sight Research Division
ATTN: Student Fellowship Program
500 East Remmington Road, Suite 200
Schaurmburg, IL 60173-4557
(847)843-2020

PHARMACOLOGY

PhRMA Foundation
ATTN: Research Fellowships
1100 15th Street, NW
Washington, DC 20005
(202)835-3400

RADIATION ONCOLOGY

Department of Radiation Oncology
ATTN: Simon Kramer Externship in
Radiation Oncology
Thomas Jefferson University Hospital
111 South 11th Street
Philadelphia, PA 19107
(215)955-5951

RHEUMATOLOGY

American College of Rheumatology
Research and Education Foundation
Medical Student Summer Clinical
Preceptorship
60 Executive Park South, Suite 150
Atlanta, GA 30329
(404)633-3777
(404)633-1870 (FAX)

UROLOGY

American Foundation for Urological Disease
ATTN: Research Scholar Division
1128 North Charles Street
Baltimore, MD 21201
(410)468-1800
(410)468-1808 (FAX)

VASCULAR SURGERY

Society for Clinical Vascular Surgery
ATTN: Essay/Research Program
13 Elm Street
Manchester, MA 01944
(508)526-8330

Appendix A

Medical School Addresses

Alabama

1. University of Alabama School of Medicine
2. University of South Alabama College of Medicine

---

1. Office of Medical Student Services/Admissions
University of Alabama School of Medicine
VH100
Birminghan, Alabama 35294-0019
(205) 934-2330
(205) 934-8724 (FAX)

2. Office of Admissions, 2015 MSB
University of South Alabama
College of Medicine
Mobile, Alabama 36688-0002
(334) 460-7176
(334) 460-6278 (FAX)

Arizona

Admissions Office, Room 2209
University of Arizona
College of Medicine
P.O. Box 245075
Tucson, Arizona 85724-5075
(520) 626-6214
(520) 626-4884 (FAX)

Arkansas

Student and Academic Affairs
University of Arkansas College of Medicine
4301 West Markham Street, Slot 551
Little Rock, Arkansas 72205-7199
(501) 686-5354
(501) 686-5873 (FAX)

California

1. University of California, Davis School of Medicine
2. University of California, Irvine College of Medicine
3. UCLA School of Medicine
4. University of California, San Diego School of Medicine
5. University of California, San Francisco School of Medicine
6. Loma Linda University School of Medicine
7. University of Southern California School of Medicine
8. Stanford University School of Medicine

---

1. Admissions Office
University of California, Davis School of Medicine
Davis, California 95616
(916) 752-2717

2. Office of Admissions and Outreach
University of California, Irvine College of Medicine
P.O. Box 4089
Medical Education Building
Irvine, California 92697-4089
(800) 824-5388 or
(714) 824-5388
(714) 824-2485 (FAX)

3. Office of Student Affairs
Division of Admissions
UCLA School of Medicine
Center for Health Sciences
Los Angeles, California 90095-1720
(310) 825-6081

4. Office of Admissions, 0621
Medical Teaching Facility
University of California, San Diego
School of Medicine
9500 Gilman Drive
La Jolla, California 92093-0621
(619) 534-3880
(619) 534-5282 (FAX)

5. School of Medicine,
   Admissions
   C-200, Box 0408
   University of California,
   San Francisco
   San Francisco, California
   94143
   (415) 476-4044

6. Associate Dean for
   Admissions
   Loma Linda University
   School of Medicine
   Loma Linda, California
   92350
   (909) 824-4467
   (909) 824-4146 (FAX)

7. Office of Admissions
   University of Southern
      California
   School of Medicine
   1975 Zonal Avenue
   (KAM 100-C)
   Los Angeles, California
   90033
   (213) 342-2552

8. Office of Admissions
   Stanford University
   School of Medicine
   851 Welch Road-Room 154
   Palo Alto, California
   94304-1677
   (415) 723-6861
   (415) 725-4599 (FAX)

Colorado

Medical School Admissions
University of Colorado
School of Medicine
4200 East 9th Avenue, C-297
Denver, Colorado 80262
(303) 315-7361
(303) 315-8494 (FAX)

Connecticut

1. University of Connecticut
   School of Medicine
2. Yale University
   School of Medicine

_____

1. Office of Admissions and
      Student Affairs
   University of Connecticut
   School of Medicine
   263 Farmington Avenue
   Rm AG-062
   Farmington, Connecticut
   06030-1905
   (860) 679-2152
   (860) 679-1282 (FAX)

2. Office of Admissions
   Yale University
   School of Medicine
   367 Cedar Street
   New Haven, Connecticut
   06510
   (203) 785-2643
   (203) 785-3234 (FAX)

Washington, D.C.

1. George Washington
   University School of
   Medicine and Health
   Sciences
2. Georgetown University
   School of Medicine
3. Howard University
   College of Medicine

_____

1. Office of Admissions
   George Washington
      University
   School of Medicine and
   Health Sciences
   2300 I Street, N.W.,
   Room 615
   Washington, D.C. 20037
   (202) 994-3506

2. Office of Admissions
   Georgetown University
   School of Medicine
   3900 Reservoir Road, N.W.
   Washington, D.C. 20007
   (202) 687-1154

3. Office of Admissions
   Office of the Dean
   Howard University
   College of Medicine
   520 W Street, N.W.
   Washington, D.C. 20059
   (202) 806-6270
   (202) 806-7934 (FAX)

Florida

1. University of Florida College of Medicine
2. University of Miami School of Medicine
3. University of South Florida College of Medicine

---

1. Chair, Medical Selection Committee
   Box 100216
   J. Hillis Miller Health Center
   University of Florida College of Medicine
   Gainesville, Florida 32610
   (352) 392-4569
   (352) 846-0622 (FAX)

2. Office of Admissions
   University of Miami School of Medicine
   P.O. Box 016159
   Miami, Florida 33101
   (305) 243-6791
   (305) 243-6548 (FAX)

3. Office of Admissions
   Box 3
   University of South Florida College of Medicine
   12901 Bruce B. Downs Boulevard
   Tampa, Florida 33612-4799
   (813) 974-2229
   (813) 974-4990 (FAX)

Georgia

1. Emory University School of Medicine
2. Medical College of Georgia School of Medicine
3. Mercer University School of Medicine
4. Morehouse School of Medicine

---

1. Medical School Admissions, Rm 303
   Woodruff Health Sciences Center
   Administration Building
   Emory University School of Medicine
   Atlanta, Georgia 30322-4510
   (404) 727-5660
   (404) 727-0045 (FAX)

2. Associate Dean for Admissions
   School of Medicine
   Medical College of Georgia
   Augusta, Georgia 30912-4760
   (706) 721-3186
   (706) 721-0959 (FAX)

3. Office of Admissions and Student Affairs
   Mercer University School of Medicine
   Macon, Georgia 31207
   (912) 752-2524
   (912) 752-2547 (FAX)

4. Admissions and Student Affairs
   Morehouse School of Medicine
   720 Westview Drive, S.W.
   Atlanta, Georgia, 30310-1495
   (404) 752-1650
   (404) 752-1512 (FAX)

Hawaii

Office of Admissions
University of Hawaii
John A. Burns School of Medicine
1960 East-West Road
Honolulu, Hawaii 96822
(808) 956-8300
(808) 956-9547 (FAX)

Illinois

1. University of Chicago Pritzker School of Medicine
2. Finch University of Health Sciences/Chicago Medical School
3. University of Illinois College of Medicine
4. Loyola University Chicago Stritch School of Medicine
5. Northwestern University Medical School
6. Rush Medical College of Rush University
7. Southern Illinois University School of Medicine

1. Office of the Dean of
   Students
   University of Chicago
   Pritzker School of
   Medicine
   924 E. 57th Street,
   BLSC 104
   Chicago, Illinois
   60637-5416
   (312) 702-1937
   (312) 702-2598 (FAX)

2. Office of Admissions
   Chicago Medical School
   3333 Green Bay Road
   North Chicago, Illinois
   60064
   (847) 578-3206/3207

3. Medical College
   Admissions
   Room 165 CME M/C 783
   University of Illinois
   College of Medicine
   808 South Wood Street
   Chicago, Illinois
   60612-7302
   (312) 996-5635
   (312) 996-6693 (FAX)

4. Loyola University Chicago
   Stritch School of Medicine
   Office of Admissions
   2160 South First Avenue
   Maywood, Illinois 60153
   (708) 216-3229

5. Northwestern University
   Medical School
   303 East Chicago Avenue
   Chicago, Illinois 60611
   (312) 503-8206

6. Office of Admissions
   524 Academic Facility
   Rush Medical College of
   Rush University
   600 South Paulina Street
   Chicago, Illinois 60612
   (312) 942-6913
   (312) 942-2333 (FAX)

7. Office of Student Affairs
   Southern Illinois
   University
   School of Medicine
   P.O. Box 19230
   Springfield, Illinois
   62794-1226
   (217) 782-2860
   (217) 785-5538 (FAX)

Indiana

Medical School Admissions
   Office
Fesler Hall 213
Indiana University
School of Medicine
1120 South Drive
Indianapolis, Indiana
46202-5113
(317) 274-3772

Iowa

Director of Admissions
University of Iowa
College of Medicine
100 Medicine Administration
   Building
Iowa City, Iowa 52242-1101
(319) 335-8052
(319) 335-8049 (FAX)

Kansas

Assistant Dean for
Admissions
University of Kansas
School of Medicine
3901 Rainbow Boulevard
Kansas City, Kansas
66160-7301
(913) 588-5245
(913) 588-5259 (FAX)

Kentucky

1. University of Kentucky
   College of Medicine
2. University of Louisville
   School of Medicine

---

1. Admissions, Room MN-102
   Office of Academic Affairs
   University of Kentucky
   College of Medicine
   Chandler Medical Center
   800 Rose Street
   Lexington, Kentucky
   40536-0084
   (606) 323-6161
   (606) 323-2076 (FAX)

2. Office of Admissions
   School of Medicine
   Health Sciences Center
   University of Louisville
   Louisville, Kentucky 40202
   (502) 852-5193

Louisiana

1. Louisiana State University
   School of Medicine in
   New Orleans
2. Louisiana State University
   Medical Center School of
   Medicine in Shreveport
3. Tulane University
   School of Medicine

---

1. Louisiana State University
   School of Medicine in
   New Orleans
   1901 Perdido Street, Box
   P3-4
   New Orleans, Louisiana
   70112-1393
   (504) 568-6262
   (504) 568-7701 (FAX)

2. Office of Student
   Admissions
   Louisiana State University
   Medical Center
   School of Medicine in
   Shreveport
   P.O. Box 33932
   Shreveport, Louisiana
   71130-3932
   (318) 675-5190
   (318) 675-5244 (FAX)

3. Office of Admissions
   Tulane University School
   of Medicine
   1430 Tulane Avenue, SL67
   New Orleans, Louisiana
   70112-2699
   (504) 588-5187
   (504) 599-6735 (FAX)

Maryland

1. Johns Hopkins University
   School of Medicine
2. University of Maryland
   School of Medicine
3. Uniformed Services
   University of the Health
   Sciences, F. Edward
   Hébert School of Medicine

---

1. Committee on Admission
   Johns Hopkins University
   School of Medicine
   720 Rutland Avenue
   Baltimore, Maryland
   21205-2196
   (410) 955-3182

2. Committee on Admissions
   Room 1-005
   University of Maryland
   School of Medicine
   655 West Baltimore Street
   Baltimore, Maryland 21201
   (410) 706-7478

3. Admissions Office
   Room A-1041
   Uniformed Services
   University
   of the Health Sciences
   F. Edward Hébert School
   of Medicine
   4301 Jones Bridge Road
   Bethesda, Maryland
   20814-4799
   (800) 772-1743 or
   (301) 295-3101
   (301) 295-3545 (FAX)

Massachusetts

1. Boston University
   School of Medicine
2. Harvard Medical School
3. University of Massachusetts
   Medical School
4. Tufts University
   School of Medicine

---

1. Admissions Office
   Building L, Room 124
   Boston University
   School of Medicine
   80 East Concord Street
   Boston, Massachusetts
   02118
   (617) 638-4630

2. Admissions Office
   Harvard Medical School
   25 Shattuck Street
   Boston, Massachusetts
   02115-6092
   (617) 432-1550
   (617) 432-3307 (FAX)

3. Associate Dean for
   Admissions
   University of
   Massachusetts Medical
   School
   55 Lake Avenue,
   NorthWorcester,
   Massachusetts 01655
   (508) 856-2323

4. Office of Admissions
   Tufts University
   School of Medicine
   136 Harrison Avenue
   Boston, Massachusetts
   02111
   (617) 636-6571

Michigan

1. Michigan State University
   College of Human
   Medicine
2. University of Michigan
   Medical School
3. Wayne State University
   School of Medicine

---

1. College of Human
   Medicine
   Office of Admissions
   A-239 Life Sciences
   Michigan State University
   East Lansing, Michigan
   48824-1317
   (517) 353-9620
   (517) 432-0021 (FAX)

2. Admissions Office
   M4130 Medical Science I
   Bldg.
   University of Michigan
   Medical School
   Ann Arbor, Michigan
   48109-0611
   (313) 764-6317
   (313) 936-3510 (FAX)

3. Director of Admissions
   Wayne State University
   School of Medicine
   540 East Canfield
   Detroit, Michigan 48201
   (313) 577-1466
   (313) 577-1330 (FAX)

Minnesota

1. Mayo Medical School
2. University of Minnesota–
   Duluth School of Medicine
3. University of Minnesota
   Medical School–
   Minneapolis

---

1. Mayo Medical School
   200 First Street, S.W.
   Rochester, Minnesota
   55905
   (507) 284-3671
   (507) 284-2634 (FAX)

2. Office of Admissions,
   Room 107
   University of Minnesota–
   Duluth
   School of Medicine
   10 University Drive
   Duluth, Minnesota 55812
   (218) 726-8511
   (218) 726-6235 (FAX)

3. University of Minnesota
   Medical School
   Office of Admissions and
   Student Affairs
   Box 293
   420 Delaware Street, S.E.
   Minneapolis, Minnesota
   55455-0310
   (612) 624-1122
   (612) 626-4200 (FAX)

Mississippi

Chairman, Admissions
   Committee
University of Mississippi
School of Medicine
2500 North State Street
Jackson, Mississippi
39216-4505
(601) 984-5010
(601) 984-5008 (FAX)

Missouri

1. University of Missouri–
   Columbia, School of
   Medicine
2. University of Missouri–
   Kansas City, School of
   Medicine

3. Saint Louis University
   School of Medicine
4. Washington University
   School of Medicine

_____

1. Office of Admissions
   MA202 Medical Sciences
     Building
   University of Missouri-
     Columbia
   School of Medicine
   One Hospital Drive
   Columbia, Missouri 65212
   (573) 882-2923
   (573) 884-4808 (FAX)

2. Council on Selection
   University of Missouri-
     Kansas City
   School of Medicine
   2411 Holmes
   Kansas City, Missouri
   64108
   (816) 235-1870
   (816) 235-5277 (FAX)

3. Admissions Committee
   Saint Louis University
   School of Medicine
   1402 South Grand
     Boulevard
   St. Louis, Missouri 63104
   (314) 577-8205
   (314) 577-8214 (FAX)

4. Office of Admissions
   Washington University
   School of Medicine
   660 South Euclid Avenue,
     #8107
   St. Louis, Missouri 63110
   (314) 362-6857
   (314) 362-4658 (FAX)

Nebraska

1. Creighton University
   School of Medicine
2. University of Nebraska
   College of Medicine

_____

1. Creighton University
   School of Medicine
   Office of Admissions
   2500 California Plaza
   Omaha, Nebraska 68178
   (402) 280-2798
   (402) 280-1241 (FAX)

2. Office of Admissions
   University of Nebraska
   College of Medicine
   Room 5017A Wittson Hall
   600 South 42nd Street
   Omaha, Nebraska
   68198-6585
   (402) 559-6140
   (402) 559-4148 (FAX)

Nevada

Office of Admissions and
  Student Affairs
University of Nevada
School of Medicine
Mail Stop 357
Reno, Nevada 89557
(702) 784-6063
(702) 784-6194 (FAX)

New Hampshire

Admissions
Dartmouth Medical School
7020 Remsen, Room 306
Hanover, New Hampshire
03755-3833
(603) 650-1505
(603) 650-1614 (FAX)

New Jersey

1. University of Medicine and
   Dentistry of New Jersey
   (UMDNJ)—New Jersey
   Medical School
2. University of Medicine and
   Dentistry of New Jersey
   (UMDNJ)—Robert Wood
   Johnson Medical School

_____

1. Director of Admissions
   UMDNJ-New Jersey
   Medical School
   185 South Orange Avenue
   Newark, New Jersey 07103
   (201) 982-4631
   (201) 982-7986 (FAX)

2. Office of Admissions
   UMDNJ-Robert Wood
   Johnson Medical School
   675 Hoes Lane
   Piscataway, New Jersey
   08854-5635
   (908) 235-4576
   (908) 235-5078 (FAX)

New Mexico

Office of Admissions and
   Student Affairs
University of New Mexico
School of Medicine
Basic Medical Sciences
   Building, Room 107
Albuquerque, New Mexico
87131-5166
(505) 277-4766
(505) 277-2755 (FAX)

New York

1. Albany Medical College
2. Albert Einstein College of
   Medicine of Yeshiva
   University
3. Columbia University
   College of Physicians and
   Surgeons
4. Cornell University Medical
   College
5. Mount Sinai School of
   Medicine
6. New York Medical College
7. New York University
   School of Medicine
8. University of Rochester
   School of Medicine and
   Dentistry

9. State University of
   New York Health Science
   Center at Brooklyn
10. State University of New
    York at Buffalo School of
    Medicine and Biomedical
    Sciences
11. SUNY Stony Brook
    School of Medicine
12. State University of New
    York Health Science
    Center at Syracuse
    College of Medicine

---

1. Office of Admissions, A-3
   Albany Medical College
   47 New Scotland Avenue
   Albany, New York 12208
   (518) 262-5521
   (518) 262-5887 (FAX)

2. Office of Admissions
   Albert Einstein College
     of Medicine of Yeshiva
     University
   Jack and Pearl Resnick
     Campus
   1300 Morris Park Avenue
   Bronx, New York 10461
   (718) 430-2106
   (718) 430-8825 (FAX)

3. Columbia University
   College of Physicians
     and Surgeons
   Admissions Office,
   Room 1-416
   630 West 168th Street
   New York, New York 10032
   (212) 305-3595

4. Office of Admissions
   Cornell University
   Medical College
   445 East 69th Street
   New York, New York 10021
   (212) 746-1067

5. Director of Admissions
   Mount Sinai School
     of Medicine
   Annenberg Building,
     Room 5-04
   One Gustave L. Levy Place-
   Box 1002
   New York, New York
   10029-6574
   (212) 241-6696

6. Office of Admissions
   Sunshine Cottage
   New York Medical College
   Valhalla, New York 10595
   (914) 993-4507
   (914) 993-4976 (FAX)

7. Office of Admissions
   New York University
   School of Medicine
   P.O. Box 1924
   New York, New York 10016
   (212) 263-5290

8. Director of Admissions
   University of Rochester
     School of Medicine and
     Dentistry
   Medical Center Box 601
   Rochester, New York 14642
   (716) 275-4539
   (716) 273-1016 (FAX)

9. Director of Admissions
State University of
New York
Health Science Center at
Brooklyn
450 Clarkson Avenue
Box 60M
Brooklyn, New York 11203
(718) 270-2446

10. Office of Medical
Admissions
University at Buffalo
40 Biomedical Education
Bldg.
Buffalo, New York
14214-3013
(716) 829-3466
(716) 829-2798 (FAX)

11. Committee on Admissions
Level 4, Room 147
Health Sciences Center
SUNY Stony Brook
School of Medicine
Stony Brook, New York
11794-8434
(516) 444-2113
(516) 444-2202 (FAX)

12. Admissions Committee
State University of New
York
Health Science Center at
Syracuse
College of Medicine
155 Elizabeth Blackwell
Street
Syracuse, New York 13210
(315) 464-4570
(315) 464-8867 (FAX)

North Carolina

1. Bowman Gray School of
Medicine of Wake Forest
University
2. Duke University School of
Medicine
3. East Carolina University
School of Medicine
4. University of North
Carolina at Chapel Hill
School of Medicine

---

1. Office of Medical School
Admissions
Bowman Gray School of
Medicine of Wake
Forest University
Medical Center Boulevard
Winston-Salem
North Carolina 27157-1090
(910) 716-4264
(910) 716-5807 (FAX)

2. Committee on Admissions
Duke University
School of Medicine
Duke University Medical
Center
P.O. Box 3710
Durham, North Carolina
27710
(919) 684-2985
(919) 684-8893 (FAX)

3. Assistant Dean
Office of Admissions
School of Medicine
East Carolina University
Greenville, North Carolina
27858-4354
(919) 816-2202

4. Admissions Office
CB# 7000 130 MacNider
Hall
University of North
Carolina at Chapel Hill
School of Medicine
Chapel Hill, North Carolina
27599-7000
(919) 962-8331

North Dakota

Secretary, Committee on
Admissions
University of North Dakota
School of Medicine and
Health Sciences
501 North Columbia Road,
Box 9037
Grand Forks, North Dakota
58202-9037
(701) 777-4221
(701) 777-4942 (FAX)

Ohio

1. Case Western Reserve
University School
of Medicine
2. University of Cincinnati
College of Medicine
3. Medical College of Ohio

4. Northeastern Ohio Universities College of Medicine
5. Ohio State University College of Medicine
6. Wright State University School of Medicine

---

1. Associate Dean for Admissions and Student Affairs
Case Western University School of Medicine
10900 Euclid Avenue
Cleveland, Ohio 44106-4920
(216) 368-3450
(216) 368-4621 (FAX)

2. Office of Student Affairs/Admissions
University of Cincinnati College of Medicine
P.O. Box 670552
Cincinnati, Ohio 45267-0552
(513) 558-7314
(513) 558-1165 (FAX)

3. Admissions Office
Medical College of Ohio
P.O. Box 10008
Toledo, Ohio 43699
(419) 381-4229
(419) 381-4005 (FAX)

4. Office of Admissions and Institutional Research
Northeastern Ohio Universities College of Medicine
P.O. Box 95
Rootstown, Ohio 44272-0095
(330) 325-2511
(330) 325-8372 (FAX)

5. Admissions Committee
270-A Meiling Hall
Ohio State University College of Medicine
370 West Ninth Avenue
Columbus, Ohio 43210-1238
(614) 292-7137
(614) 292-1544 (FAX)

6. Office of Student Affairs/Admissions
Wright State University School of Medicine
P.O. Box 1751
Dayton, Ohio 45401
(937) 775-2934
(937) 775-3322 (FAX)

Oklahoma

University of Oklahoma College of Medicine
P.O. Box 26901
Oklahoma City, Oklahoma 73190
(405) 271-2331
(405) 271-3032 (FAX)

Oregon

Office of Education and Student Affairs, L102
Oregon Health Sciences University
3181 S.W. Sam Jackson Park Road
Portland, Oregon 97201
(503) 494-2998
(503) 494-3400 (FAX)

Pennsylvania

1. Allegheny University of the Health Sciences: Medical College of Pennsylvania/ Hahnemann School of Medicine
2. Jefferson Medical College of Thomas Jefferson University
3. Pennsylvania State University College of Medicine
4. University of Pennsylvania School of Medicine
5. University of Pittsburgh School of Medicine
6. Temple University School of Medicine

---

1. Admissions Office
MCP/Hahnemann School of Medicine
2900 Queen Lane Avenue
Philadelphia, Pennsylvania 19129
(215) 991-8202
(215) 843-1766 (FAX)

2. Associate Dean for
   Admissions
   Jefferson Medical College
   of Thomas Jefferson
   University
   1025 Walnut Street
   Philadelphia, Pennsylvania
   19107
   (215) 955-6983
   (215) 923-6939 (FAX)

3. Office of Student Affairs
   Pennsylvania State
   University
   College of Medicine
   P.O. Box 850
   Hershey, Pennsylvania
   17033
   (717) 531-8755
   (717) 531-6225 (FAX)

4. Director of Admissions and
   Financial Aid
   Edward J. Stemmler Hall,
   Suite 100
   University of Pennsylvania
   School of Medicine
   Philadelphia, Pennsylvania
   19104-6056
   (215) 898-8001
   (215) 573-6645 (FAX)

5. Office of Admissions
   518 Scaife Hall
   University of Pittsburgh
   School of Medicine
   Pittsburgh, Pennsylvania
   15261
   (412) 648-9891
   (412) 648-8768 (FAX)

6. Admissions Office
   Suite 305
   Student Faculty Center
   Temple University
   School of Medicine
   Broad and Ontario Streets
   Philadelphia, Pennsylvania
   19140
   (215) 707-3656
   (215) 707-6932 (FAX)

Puerto Rico

1. Universidad Central del
   Caribe School of Medicine
2. Ponce School of Medicine
3. University of Puerto Rico
   School of Medicine

---

1. Office of Admissions
   Universidad Central del
   Caribe
   School of Medicine
   Call Box 60-327
   Bayamón, Puerto Rico
   00960-6032
   (787) 740-1611 Ext. 210
   (787) 269-7550 (FAX)

2. Admissions Office
   Ponce School of Medicine
   P.O. Box 7004
   Ponce, Puerto Rico 00732
   (787) 840-2511
   (787) 844-3685 (FAX)

3. Central Admissions Office
   School of Medicine
   Medical Sciences Campus
   University of Puerto Rico
   P.O. Box 365067
   San Juan, Puerto Rico
   00936-5067
   (787) 758-2525 Ext. 5213
   (787) 282-7117 (FAX)

Rhode Island

Office of Admissions and
   Financial Aid
Brown University
School of Medicine
97 Waterman Street,
   Box G-A212
Providence, Rhode Island
   02912-9706
(401) 863-2149
(401) 863-2660 (FAX)

South Carolina

1. Medical University of
   South Carolina
2. University of South
   Carolina School of
   Medicine

---

1. Office of Enrollment
   Services
   Medical University of
   South Carolina
   171 Ashley Avenue
   Charleston, South Carolina
   29425
   (803) 792-3281
   (803) 792-3764 (FAX)

2. Associate Dean for Medical Education and Academic Affairs
University of South Carolina School of Medicine
Columbia, South Carolina 29208
(803) 733-3325
(803) 733-3328 (FAX)

South Dakota

Office of Student Affairs, Room 105
University Of South Dakota School of Medicine
414 East Clark Street
Vermillion, South Dakota 57069-2390
(605) 677-5233
(605) 677-5109 (FAX)

Tennessee

1. East Tennessee State University James H. Quillen College of Medicine
2. Meharry Medical College
3. University of Tennessee, Memphis College of Medicine
4. Vanderbilt University School of Medicine

1. Assistant Dean for Admissions and Records
East Tennessee State University
James H. Quillen College of Medicine
P.O. Box 70580
Johnson City, Tennessee 37614-0580
(423) 439-6221
(423) 439-6616 (FAX)

2. Director, Admissions and Records
Meharry Medical College
1005 D.B. Todd Boulevard
Nashville, Tennessee 37208
(615) 327-6223
(615) 327-6228 (FAX)

3. University of Tennessee, Memphis
College of Medicine
790 Madison Avenue
Memphis, Tennessee 38163-2166
(901) 448-5559
(901) 448-7255 (FAX)

4. Office of Admissions
209 Light Hall
Vanderbilt University School of Medicine
Nashville, Tennessee 37232-0685
(615) 322-2145
(615) 343-8397 (FAX)

Texas

1. Baylor College of Medicine
2. Texas A&M University Health Science Center College of Medicine
3. Texas Tech University School of Medicine
4. University of Texas Southwestern Medical Center at Dallas
5. University of Texas Medical Branch at Galveston School of Medicine
6. University of Texas– Houston Medical School
7. University of Texas Health Science Center at San Antonio

1. Office of Admissions
Baylor College of Medicine
One Baylor Plaza
Houston, Texas 77030
(713) 798-4842

2. Director of Admissions
Texas A&M University Health Science Center College of Medicine
College Station, Texas 77843-1114
(409) 845-7744
(409) 847-8663 (FAX)

3. Office of Admissions
   Texas Tech University
   Health Sciences Center
   School of Medicine
   Lubbock, Texas 79430
   (806) 743-2297
   (806) 743-3021 (FAX)

4. Office of the Registrar
   University of Texas
   Southwestern Medical
   Center at Dallas
   5323 Harry Hines
   Boulevard
   Dallas, Texas 75235-9096
   (214) 648-2670
   (214) 648-3289 (FAX)

5. Office of Admissions
   G-210, Ashbel Smith
   Building
   University of Texas
   Medical Branch at
   Galveston
   School of Medicine
   Galveston, Texas
   77555-1317
   (409) 772-3517
   (409) 772-5753 (FAX)

6. Office of Admissions-
   Room G-024
   University of Texas–
   Houston Medical School
   P.O. Box 20708
   Houston, Texas 77225
   (713) 500-5116
   (713) 500-0604 (FAX)

7. Medical School Admissions
   Registrar's Office
   University of Texas
   Health Science Center at
   San Antonio
   7703 Floyd Curl Drive
   San Antonio, Texas
   78284-7701
   (210) 567-2665
   (210) 567-2685 (FAX)

Utah

Director of Medical School
   Admissions
University of Utah
School of Medicine
50 North Medical Drive
Salt Lake City, Utah 84132
(801) 581-7498
(801) 585-3300 (FAX)

Vermont

Admissions Office
C-225 Given Building
University of Vermont
College of Medicine
Burlington, Vermont 05405
(802) 656-2154

Virginia

1. Eastern Virginia Medical
   School
2. Virginia Commonwealth
   University-Medical College
   of Virginia School of
   Medicine
3. University of Virginia
   School of Medicine

1. Office of Admissions
   Eastern Virginia Medical
   School
   721 Fairfax Avenue
   Norfolk, Virginia
   23507-2000
   (757) 446-5812
   (757) 446-5896 (FAX)

2. Virginia Commonwealth
   University
   Medical College of
   Virginia   School of
   Medicine
   P.O. Box 980565
   Richmond, Virginia
   23298-0565
   (804) 828-9629
   (804) 828-1246 (FAX)

3. Medical School Admissions
   Office
   Box 235
   University of Virginia
   School of Medicine
   Charlottesville, Virginia
   22908
   (804) 924-5571
   (804) 982-2586 (FAX)

Washington

Admissions Ofice
Health Sciences Center A-300
Box 356340
University of Washington
Seattle, Washington
98195-6340
(206) 543-7212

West Virginia

1. Marshall University School of Medicine
2. West Virginia University Health Sciences Center

---

1. Admissions Office
   Marshall University
   School of Medicine
   1542 Spring Valley Drive
   Huntington, West Virginia 25704
   (800) 544-8514 or
   (304) 696-7312

2. Office of Admissions and Records
   West Virginia University
   Health Sciences Center
   P.O. Box 9815
   Morgantown, West Virginia 26506
   (304) 293-3521
   (304) 293-7968 (FAX)

Wisconsin

1. Medical College of Wisconsin
2. University of Wisconsin Medical School

1. Office of Admissions and Registrar
   Medical College of Wisconsin
   8701 Watertown Plank Road
   Milwaukee, Wisconsin 53226
   (414) 456-8246

2. Admissions Committee
   Medical Sciences Center
   Room1140
   University of Wisconsin
   Medical School
   1300 University Avenue
   Madison, Wisconsin 53706
   (608) 263-4925
   (608) 262-2327 (FAX)

Appendix B

Abbreviations Commonly Used In
The Premedical/Medical School Literature

AACOM:	American Association of Colleges of Osteopathic Medicine
AACOMAS:	American Association of Colleges of Osteopathic Medicine Application Service
AAMC:	Association of American Medical Colleges
ACGME:	Accreditation Council for Graduate Medical Education
ACT:	American College Testing Program
AMA:	American Medical Association
AMCAS:	American Medical College Application Service
AMCAS-E:	American Medical College Application Service (Electronic)
AMSA:	American Medical Student Association
AMWA:	American Medical Women's Association
AOA:	American Osteopathic Association
AP:	Advanced Placement
CLEP:	College Level Examination Program
CSA:	Clinical Skills Assessment
D.O.:	Doctor of Osteopathic Medicine/Doctor of Osteopathy
ECFMG:	Educational Commission for Foreign Medical Graduates
EDP:	Early Decision Plan
ENT:	Ear, Nose, and Throat (Otolaryngology)
FMG:	Foreign Medical Graduate
GPA:	Grade Point Average
GRE:	Graduate Record Examination
HMO:	Health Maintenance Organization
IMG:	International Medical Graduate
INMED:	Indians Into Medicine Program
LCME:	Liaison Committee on Medical Education
M.D.:	Medical Doctor/Doctor of Medicine
M.B.A.:	Master of Business Administration
MCAT:	Medical College Admission Test

Sections on the MCAT

BS: Biological Sciences

PS: Physical Sciences

VR: Verbal Reasoning

WS: Writing Sample

M.H.A.:   Master of Health Administration

MMEP: Minority Medical Education Program

M.P.H.:   Master of Public Health

MSTP: Medical Scientist Training Program
(M.D./Ph.D. Program)

NBME: National Board of Medical Examiners

NBOME: National Board of Osteopathic Medical Examiners

NIH: National Institutes of Health

NPSA: National Prehealth Student Association

OMM: Osteopathic Manipulative Medicine

OMCAS: Ontario Medical School Application Service

PBL: Problem Based Learning

PGY: Post-Graduate Year

PH.D.:   Doctor of Philosophy

RRC: Residency Review Committee

SAT: Scholastic Aptitude Test

SOMA: Student Osteopathic Medical Association

USIMG: United States International Medical Graduate

USMLE: United States Medical Licensing Examination

WAMI: Washington, Alaska, Montana, Idaho

WHO: World Health Organization

WICHE: Western Interstate Commission for Higher Education

Appendix C

Examples of Medical/Surgical Specialties, Subspecialties and/or Fellowship Training

1. Examples of Specialties

Aerospace Medicine	Orthopaedic Surgery
Allergy and Immunology	Otolaryngology
Anesthesiology	Pathology
Colon and Rectal Surgery	Pediatrics
Dermatology	Physical Medicine and Rehabilitation
Emergency Medicine	Plastic Surgery
Family Practice	Preventive Medicine
Internal Medicine	Psychiatry
Medical Genetics	Radiology (Diagnostic)
Neurological Surgery	Radiation Oncology
Neurology	Surgery (General)
Nuclear Medicine	Thoracic Surgery
Obstetrics and Gynecology	Urology
Ophthalmology	

It is important to note that many specialties will require one or more years of preliminary training in general medicine or general surgery. With some disciplines, resident physicians do not "jump right into their specialty" but take a year of internal medicine or general surgery or a "transitional year" which covers areas such as internal medicine, surgery, OB/GYN, pediatrics, the intensive care unit, the emergency room, and other electives. Though every specialty will not be discussed, a few examples will be given to provide the reader with a general overview of preliminary training requirements. (Note: The American Medical Association publishes the *Graduate Medical Education Directory* (updated annually) which provides information on specialty training programs and their requirements. This directory also includes the programs accredited by the Accreditation Council for Graduate Medical Education [ACGME].)

Some specialties require a firm foundation in clinical based medicine. For example, many resident physicians in the areas of emergency medicine, dermatology, anesthesiology, ophthalmology, and physical medicine and rehabilitation fulfill this requirement by taking a year of internal medicine before beginning specialty training. With surgical specialties such as orthopaedics, neurosurgery, and plastic surgery, at least one year of general surgery is required before proceeding with further training. Some specialties (*e.g.* physical medicine and rehabilitation, ophthalmology) may allow the resident physician to fulfill their first year of postgraduate training (PGY-1) with a "transitional year" (with an emphasis on developing good clinical skills).

The following list gives examples of subspecialty and/or fellowship training in some of the areas of medicine and surgery. Additional expertise in a chosen field does require the physician to extend his/her training period. The time duration will depend on the specialty/subspecialty/fellowship. (*e.g.* A cardiologist must complete a three year internal medicine residency before training in cardiology for an additional three years). This listing does not have every possible subspecialty/fellowship but is used only to exemplify some of the areas of expertise which need additional training beyond the basic residency period.

2. Examples of Subspecialty/Fellowship Training

- Allergy and Immunology
    - Clinical and Laboratory Immunology

- Anesthesiology
    - Critical Care Medicine
    - Pain Management

- Dermatology
    - Dermatopathology

- Emergency Medicine
    - Sports Medicine

- Family Practice
    - Geriatric Medicine
    - Sports Medicine

- Internal Medicine
    - *e.g.* Cardiovascular Disease (Cardiology)
    - Critical Care Medicine
    - Endocrinology
    - Gastroenterology
    - Hematology
    - Pulmonary Disease
    - Rheumatology

- Neurological Surgery
    - Pediatric Neurological Surgery

- Neurology
    - Child Neurology

- Obstetrics and Gynecology
    - Gynecologic Oncology
    - Maternal/Fetal Medicine
    - Oncology
    - Reproductive Endocrinology
    - Urogynecology

- Ophthalmology
  e.g. Neuro-ophthalmology
    Diseases of the Retina

- Orthopaedic Surgery
  e.g. Hand Surgery
    Orthopaedic Trauma
    Pediatric Orthopaedics

- Otolaryngology
    Otology/Neurotology
    Pediatric Otolaryngology

- Pathology
  e.g. Blood Banking/Transfusion Medicine
    Forensic Pathology
    Neuropathology

- Pediatrics
  e.g. Pediatric Cardiology
    Pediatric Critical Care Medicine
    Pediatric Hematology/Oncology
    Pediatric Pulmonology

- Physical Medicine and Rehabilitation
    Spinal Cord Injury Medicine

- Plastic Surgery
    Hand Surgery

- Psychiatry
  e.g. Child and Adolescent Psychiatry
    Forensic Psychiatry
    Geriatric Psychiatry

- Radiology/Diagnostic
  e.g. Neuroradiology
    Pediatric Radiology

- Surgery
    Surgical Critical Care
    Pediatric Surgery
    Vascular Surgery

- Urology
    Pediatric Urology

3. List of Medical Specialty Contacts

(Note: The organizations marked with an asterisk (*) provide additional information [*e.g.* brochures, pamphlets, etc.] to those who are considering that specialty as a profession.)

AEROSPACE MEDICINE

* Aerospace Medical Association
  320 South Henry Street
  Alexandria, VA 22314-3579
  (703)739-2240
  (703)739-9652 (FAX)

ALLERGY AND IMMUNOLOGY

1. American Academy of Allergy,
  Asthma, and Immunology
  611 East Wells Street
  Milwaukee, WI 53202
  (414)272-6071
  (414)272-6070 (FAX)

2. American College of Allergy,
   Asthma, and Immunology
   85 West Algonquin Road, Suite 550
   Arlington Heights, IL 60005
   (847)427-1200
   (847)427-1294 (FAX)

ANESTHESIOLOGY

* American Society of Anesthesiologists
  520 North Northwest Highway
  Park Ridge, IL 60068
  (847)825-5586
  (847)825-1692 (FAX)

CARDIOLOGY

  American College of Cardiology
  9111 Old Georgetown Road
  Bethesda, MD 20814
  (301)897-2622
  (301)897-9745 (FAX)

COLON AND RECTAL SURGERY

* American Society of Colon and
  Rectal Surgeons
  85 West Algonquin Road, Suite 550
  Arlington Heights, IL 60005
  (847)290-9184
  (847)290-9203 (FAX)

CRITICAL CARE MEDICINE

  Society of Critical Care Medicine
  8101 East Kaiser Boulevard
  Anaheim, CA 92808-2214
  (714)282-6000
  (714)282-6050 (FAX)

DERMATOLOGY

* American Academy of Dermatology
  PO Box 4014
  Schaumburg, IL 60168-4014
  (847)330-0230
  (847)330-0050 (FAX)

EMERGENCY MEDICINE

  American College of Emergency Physicians
  PO Box 619911
  Dallas, TX 75261-9911
  (972)550-0911
  (972)580-2816 (FAX)

FAMILY PRACTICE

* American Academy of Family Physicians
  8880 Ward Parkway
  Kansas City, MO 64114
  (816)333-9700
  (816)822-0580 (FAX)

GERIATRIC MEDICINE

  American Geriatrics Society
  770 Lexington Avenue, Suite 300
  New York, NY 10021
  (212)308-1414
  (212)832-8646 (FAX)

INTERNAL MEDICINE

* American Society of Internal Medicine
  2011 Pennsylvania Avenue, NW, Ste 800
  Washington, DC 20006-1808
  (202)835-2746
  (202)835-0443 (FAX)

NEUROLOGICAL SURGERY

1. Neurosurgical Society of America
   UCLA Division of Neurosurgery
   10833 Le Conte Avenue
   Los Angeles, CA 90024
   (310)825-3998
   (310)794-2147 (FAX)

2. Society of Neurological Surgeons
   New England Medical Center
   Department of Neurosurgery
   750 Washington Street
   PO Box 178
   Boston, MA 02111
   (617)636-5858

NEUROLOGY

* 1. American Academy of Neurology
   2221 University Avenue, SE, Suite 335
   Minneapolis, MN 55414
   (612)623-8115
   (612)623-2491 (FAX)

2. American Neurological Association
   5841 Cedar Lake Road, Suite 108
   Minneapolis, MN 55416
   (612)545-6284
   (612)545-6073 (FAX)

NUCLEAR MEDICINE

Society of Nuclear Medicine
1850 Samuel Morse Drive
Reston, VA 22090
(703)708-9000
(703)708-9015 (FAX)

OBSTETRICS AND GYNECOLOGY

1. American College of Obstetricians
   and Gynecologists
   409 12th Street, SW
   Washington, DC 20024-2188
   (202)638-5577
   (202)484-5107 (FAX)

2. American Society for Reproductive
   Medicine
   1209 Montgomery Highway
   Birmingham, AL 35216-2809
   (205)978-5000
   (205)978-5005 (FAX)

OCCUPATIONAL AND ENVIRONMENTAL MEDICINE

1. American Academy of
   Environmental Medicine
   4510 West 89th Street, Suite 110
   Prairie Village, KS 66207-2282
   (913)642-6062
   (913)341-6912 (FAX)

2. American College of Occupational and
   Environmental Medicine
   55 West Seegers
   Arlington Heights, IL 60005
   (847)228-6850
   (847)228-1856 (FAX)

ONCOLOGY

1. American Society of Clinical Oncology
   225 Reinekers Lane
   Suite 650
   Alexandria, VA 22314
   (703) 299-0150
   (703) 299-1044 (FAX)

2. American Society for Therapeutic
   Radiology and Oncology
   1891 Preston White Drive
   Reston, VA 22091
   (800) 962-7876
   (703) 476-8167 (FAX)

3. Society of Surgical Oncology
   85 West Algonquin Road
   Suite 550
   Arlington Heights, IL 60005
   (847) 427-1400
   (847) 427-9656 (FAX)

OPHTHALMOLOGY

* 1. American Academy of Ophthalmology
   655 Beach Street
   PO Box 7424
   San Francisco, CA 94120
   (415) 561-8500
   (415) 561-8533 (FAX)

2. American Ophthalmological Society
   Duke University Eye Center
   Box 3802
   Durham, NC 27710-3802
   (919) 684-5365
   (919) 684-2230 (FAX)

ORTHOPAEDIC SURGERY

* 1. American Academy of Orthopaedic
   Surgeons
   6300 North River Road
   Rosemont, IL 60018-4262
   (847) 823-7186
   (847) 823-8125 (FAX)

2. The American Orthopaedic Association
   6300 North River Road, Suite 300
   Rosemont, IL 60018-4263
   (847) 318-7330
   (847) 318-7339 (FAX)

3. American College of Foot
   and Ankle Surgeons
   515 Busse Highway
   Park Ridge, IL 60068
   (847) 292-2237
   (847) 292-2022 (FAX)

OTOLARYNGOLOGY

1. American Academy of Otolaryngology-
   Head and Neck Surgery, Inc.
   One Prince Street
   Alexandria, VA 22314
   (703) 836-4444
   (703) 683-5100 (FAX)

2. American Otological Society, Inc.
   Loyola University Medical Center
   2160 South First Avenue
   Building 105, Number 1870
   Maywood, IL 60153
   (708) 216-8526
   (708) 216-4834 (FAX)

3. American Society for Head and
   Neck Surgery
   203 Lothrop Street, Suite 250
   Pittsburgh, PA 15213
   (410) 955-7400

* 4. Society of University Otolaryngologists
   Head and Neck Surgeons
   Joint Center for Otolaryngology
   Harvard Medical School
   333 Longwood Avenue
   Boston, MA 02115
   (617) 732-7003
   (617) 217-1372 (FAX)

PATHOLOGY

1. American Society of Clinical Pathologists
   2100 West Harrison Street
   Chicago, IL 60612-3798
   (312) 738-1336
   (312) 738-9798 (FAX)

* 2. College of American Pathologists
   325 Waukegan Road
   Northfield, IL 60093-2750
   (800) 323-4040 or
   (847) 832-7000
   (847) 832-8151 (FAX)

3. Intersociety Committee on Pathology
   Information, Inc.
   4733 Bethesda, MD 20814
   (301) 656-2944

PEDIATRICS

* 1. American Academy of Pediatrics
   141 Northwest Point Boulevard
   PO Box 927
   Elk Grove Village, IL 60009-0927
   (847) 228-5005
   (847) 228-5097 (FAX)

2. American Pediatric Society, Inc.
   141 Northwest Point Boulevard
   PO Box 675
   Elk Grove Village, IL 60009-0675
   (847) 427-0205
   (847) 427-1305 (FAX)

PHYSICAL MEDICINE AND REHABILITATION

1. American Academy of Physical
   Medicine and Rehabilitation
   One IBM Plaza, Suite 2500
   Chicago, IL 60611-3604
   (312) 464-9700
   (312) 464-0227 (FAX)

* 2. Association of Academic Physiatrists
   5987 East 71st Street, Suite 112
   Indianapolis, IN 46220
   (317) 845-4200

PLASTIC SURGERY

1. American Academy of Facial Plastic
   and Reconstructive Surgery, Inc.
   1110 Vermont Avenue, NW
   Suite 220
   Washington, DC 20005
   (202) 842-4500
   (202) 371-1514 (FAX)

2. American Association of Plastic
Surgeons
2317 Seminole Road
Atlantic Beach, FL 32233
(904)359-3759
(904)359-3789 (FAX)

3. American Society of Plastic and
Reconstructive Surgeons
444 East Algonquin Road
Arlington, Heights, IL 60005
(847)228-9900
(847)228-9131 (FAX)

PREVENTIVE MEDICINE

American College of Preventive Medicine
1660 L Street, NW
Washington, DC 20036
(202)466-2044
(202)466-2662 (FAX)

PUBLIC HEALTH

American Association of Public Health
Physicians
Department of Preventive Medicine and
Public Health
1600 Canal Street
New Orleans, LA 70112
(504)568-6935
(504)568-6905 (FAX)

PULMONOLOGY

American College of Chest Physicians
3300 Dundee Road
Northbrook, IL 60062-2348
(847)498-1400
(847)498-5460 (FAX)

PSYCHIATRY

* 1. American Psychiatric Association
1400 K Street, NW
Washington, DC 20005
(202)682-6000
(202)682-6114 (FAX)

2. American Association for Geriatric
Psychiatry
7910 Woodmont Avenue
Seventh Floor
Bethesda, MD 20814-3004
(301)654-7850
(301)654-4137 (FAX)

* 3. American Academy of Child and
Adolescent Psychiatry
3615 Wisconsin Avenue, NW
Washington, DC 20016
(202)966-7300
(202)966-2891 (FAX)

4. American Society for Adolescent
Psychiatry
4340 East West Highway, Suite 401
Bethesda, MD 20814
(301)718-6502
(301)656-0989 (FAX)

RADIOLOGY

* American College of Radiology
1891 Preston White Drive
Reston, VA 20191-4397
(703)648-8900
(703)648-9176 (FAX)

RHEUMATOLOGY

American College of Rheumatology
60 Executive Park South, Suite 150
Atlanta, GA 30329
(404)633-3777
(404)633-1870 (FAX)

SPORTS MEDICINE

* 1. American College of Sports Medicine
PO Box 1440
Indianapolis, IN 46206-1440
(317)637-9200
(317)634-7817 (FAX)

2. The American Orthopaedic Society
for Sports Medicine
6300 N. River Road, Suite 200
Rosemont, IL 60018
(708)292-4900
(708)292-4905 (FAX)

SURGERY

1. American Association for the
Surgery of Trauma
Harborview Medical Center
AAST/Department of Surgery
325 Ninth Avenue, Box 359796
Seattle, WA 98104-2499
(206)731-3299
(206)731-8582 (FAX)

* 2. American College of Surgeons
55 East Erie Street
Chicago, IL 60611
(312)664-4050
(312)440-7014 (FAX)

3. American Surgical Association
13 Elm Street
Manchester, MA 01944
(508)526-8330
(508)526-4018 (FAX)

THORACIC SURGERY

American Thoracic Society
1740 Broadway
New York, NY 10019-4374
(212)315-8700
(212)315-6498 (FAX)

UROLOGY

American Urological Association, Inc.
1120 North Charles Street
Baltimore, MD 21201
(410)223-4300
(410)223-4370 (FAX)

Appendix D

Information Resource Addresses

Applications

MCAT Program Office
2255 North Dubuque Road
PO Box 4056
Iowa City, IA 52243-4056
(319) 337-1357
(319) 337-1122 (FAX)

Additional Score Reports
Section for Student Services
Association of American Medical Colleges
2501 M Street, NW, Suite 1
Washington, DC 20037-1300

American Medical College Application
Service (AMCAS)
Association of American Medical Colleges
Section for Student Services
2501 M Street, NW, Lobby-26
Washington, DC 20037-1300
(202) 828-0600

American Association of Colleges of
Osteopathic Medicine Application Service
(AACOMAS)
5550 Friendship Boulevard, Suite 310
Chevy Chase, MD 20815-7231
(301) 968-4190

University of Texas System Medical
Application Center
702 Colorado, Suite 620
Austin, TX 78712
(512) 475-7399
(512) 555-1212 (FAX)

Licensing

Federation of State Medical Boards of
the United States, Inc.
Federation Place
400 Fuller Wiser Road, Suite 300
Euless, TX 76039-3855
(817) 868-4000

MD/Ph.D. Programs

Program Administrator
Medical Scientist Training Program
National Institutes of Health
45 Center Drive, MSC 6200
Bethesda, MD 20892-6200
(301) 594-3830

Medical Schools

Association of American Medical Colleges
2450 N Street, NW
Washington, DC 20037-1127
(202) 828-0400
(202) 828-1125 (FAX)

Membership and Publication Orders
Association of American Medical Colleges
2450 N Street, NW
Washington, DC 20037-1129
(202) 828-1123

AMCAS
Association of American Medical Colleges
Section for Student Services
2501 M Street, NW
Washington, DC 20037-1127
(202) 828-0600

Medical Specialties/Education

National Board of Medical Examiners
ATTN: USMLE
3750 Market Street
Philadelphia, PA 19104
(215) 590-9500
(215) 590-9755 (FAX)

Council of Medical Specialties Societies
51 Sherwood Terrace, Suite Y
Lake Bluff, IL 60044-2202
(847) 295-3456
(847) 295-3759 (FAX)

National Resident Matching Program
(NRMP)
2501 M Street, NW, Suite 1
Washington, DC 20037-1307
(202) 828-0676

Committee of Interns and Residents
386 Park Avenue, S
New York, NY 10016
(212) 725-5500
(212) 779-2413 (FAX)

American Board of Medical Specialties
(ABMS)
1007 Church Street, Suite 404
Evanston, IL 60201-5913
(847) 491-9091
(847) 328-3596 (FAX)

Accreditation Council for Graduate Medical
Education (ACGME)
515 North State Street, Suite 2000
Chicago, IL 60610
(312) 464-4920
(312) 464-4098 (FAX)

Association of Academic Health Centers
1400 Sixteenth Street, NW, Suite 720
Washington, DC 20036
(202) 265-9600
(202) 265-7514 (FAX)

Association for Hospital Medical Education
1200 19th Street, NW, Suite 300
Washington, DC 20036-2422
(202) 857-1196
(202) 223-4579 (FAX)

Educational Commission for Foreign
Medical Graduates (ECFMG)
3624 Market Street
Philadelphia, PA 19104-2685
(215) 386-5900
(215) 387-9963 (FAX)

Medical Students

The American Medical Students
Association/Foundation
1902 Association Drive
Reston, VA 22091
(703) 620-6600
(703) 620-5873 (FAX)

Minority Students

Minority Student Information
Clearinghouse
Division of Community and Minority
Programs
Association of American Medical Colleges
2450 N Street, NW
Washington, DC 20037-1126

Student National Medical Association
1012 Tenth Street, NW
Washington, DC 20001
(202) 371-1616
(202) 371-5676 (FAX)

Minority Medical Education Program
Association of American Medical Colleges
Section for Student Services
2501 M Street, NW, Lobby-26
Washington, DC 20037-1300
(202) 828- 0400
(202) 828-1124 (FAX)
Office of Statewide Health Planning and
Development
Health Profession Career Opportunity
Program
1600 Ninth Street, Room 441
Sacramento, CA 95814
(916) 654-1730

Osteopathic Medicine

American Association of Colleges of
Osteopathic Medicine
5550 Friendship Boulevard, Suite 310
Chevy Chase, MD 20815
(301) 968-4100
(301) 968-4101 (FAX)

The American Osteopathic Association
142 East Ontario Street
Chicago, IL 60611
(312) 280-5800
(312) 280-3860 (FAX)

The American Academy of Osteopathy
3500 DePauw Boulevard, Suite 1080
Indianapolis, IN 46268-1136
(317) 879-1881
(317) 879-0563

American Osteopathic
Healthcare Association
5301 Wisconsin Avenue, NW, Suite 630
Washington, DC 20015
(202) 686-1700
(202) 686-7615 (FAX)

Women in Medicine

Staff, Women in Medicine Program
Division of Institutional Planning
and Development
Association of American Medical Colleges
2450 N Street, NW
Washington, DC 20037-1126

AMA Women in Medicine Services
Women and Minority Services
515 North State Street
Chicago, IL 60610
(312) 464-4392
(312) 464-5845 (FAX)

National Osteopathic Women Physicians
Association
5301 Wisconsin Avenue, NW
Suite 630
Washington, DC 20015
(202) 686-1700
(202) 537-1362 (FAX)

Financial Aid Resources for Women

American Fellowships and Selected
Profession Fellowships
American Association Foundation of
University Women (AAUW)
Educational Foundation
2201 North Dodge Street
PO Box 4030
Iowa City, IA 52243-4030
(319) 337-1716
(319) 337-1204 (FAX)

Business and Professional Women's
Foundation Scholarship Program
2012 Massachusetts Avenue, NW
Washington, DC 20036

American Medical Women's Association
(AMWA)
Medical Education Loan Program
800 North Fairfax Street
Suite 400
Alexandria, VA 22314
(703) 838-0500
(703) 549-3864 (FAX)

Other

Professional Student Exchange Program
Western Interstate Commission for Higher
Education (WICHE)
PO Drawer P
Boulder, CO 80301-9752
(303) 541-0214

Index

Notes

Notes

Notes